Living Sensationally

"Dr. Winnie Dunn has solved one of the great mysteries of life—the sensory puzzle! This amazing book helps everyone understand their sensory systems and thereby improves quality of life. This book is essential for anyone who wants to understand themselves and their family, friends, and community."

—Brenda Smith Myles, University of Kansas, USA

"Life is full of different sensations—we cannot escape them so why not delight in our daily sensory experiences! Using up to date research information, Winnie Dunn leads the reader through a personal discovery process about their sensory experiences. Through practical examples, you will learn how to live each day to match your activities with your sensory needs. The result can be educational, fun and fulfilling!"

—Mary Law, Professor and Associate Dean of Rehabilitation Science, McMaster University, Ontario, Canada

"Dr. Dunn's work on sensory systems has been a critical link in understanding the issues of children with attention deficits and autism; she has now written the book that all of us can use to understand how our sensory systems and our sensory preferences define us as individuals."

—Carolyn Baum, Professor of Occupational Therapy and Neurology, Washington University, USA

Living Sensationally

Understanding Your Senses

Winnie Dunn

Jessica Kingsley Publishers
London and Philadelphia

Quote from *City of Angels* on p.24 reproduced with kind permission from
Warner Bros. Entertainment Inc.

First published in 2008
by Jessica Kingsley Publishers
116 Pentonville Road
London N1 9JB, UK
and
400 Market Street, Suite 400
Philadelphia, PA 19106, USA

www.jkp.com

Library of Congress Cataloging in Publication Data

Dunn, Winnie.

Living sensationally : understanding your senses / Winnie Dunn.

p. cm.

Includes bibliographical references.

ISBN-13: 978-1-84310-871-9 (pbk. : alk. paper) 1. Senses and sensation. I. Title.

BF233.D86 2008

152.1—dc22

2007019751

British Library Cataloguing in Publication Data

A CIP catalogue record for this book is available from the British Library

ISBN 978 1 84310 871 9

Printed and bound in the United States by
Thomson-Shore, Inc.

To Andrew Timothy Wilson, my husband.
What more could a Seeker like me ask for
but a loving, kind, accepting Bystander like him?

Contents

Tables

Preface

What does a guy who still hears the "silent" garage door opener have to do with you?

In my research, I have identified some patterns of human behavior. Specifically, people have different ways of reacting to sensory experiences in their everyday lives. The reactions can be more easily understood when we study people whose sensory processing is so unusual that it interferes with even desirable life activities; people with disorders such as Asperger's syndrome, autism, Attention Deficit Disorder, and learning disabilities can have these unusual sensory processing patterns. The concepts involved are not as clear when studying people without particular disorders because most people have moderate behaviors that don't stand out. People with disorders that include unusual sensory processing patterns live a more intense version of life; they experience things more acutely or more deeply. The intensity of their experiences can be informative to the rest of us because our more moderate responses could go unnoticed, even though understanding the meaning of our behaviors can be very helpful.

I have realized from my research that everyone's behavior is on a continuum. This book makes my research available to all people so they can understand themselves, their family members, friends, and co-workers a little better. People with disorders have an important gift to give. They give us insight about what our own responses might mean because they experience amplified versions of life. When we begin to understand that everyone's behaviors are on the same continuum of responses, it is easier to see we are more like each other than different from each other. This book enables all of us to understand the nature of our individual differences (particularly in relation to our responses to sensory experiences), which in turn makes us more interesting to each other. You may know the guy with the silent garage door opener, and this book will help you understand his need for quiet, making your relationship more successful and satisfying for both of you.

Acknowledgements

During the formative stages of developing this book, an incredible group of friends agreed to meet once a month for an entire year to discuss ideas with each other. I would send out something I had written that month, and the group would discuss their reactions to the material. I took notes and *listened*. I called this time our *Sensational Conversations* (SC).

At first I wrote essays, short descriptions, explanations, and stories. As my SC group grew in wisdom and insights, essays turned into chapters, and stories took shape as clear, crisp examples of the power of sensory input in people's lives. These friends continue to talk about sensation and have offered me countless stories from their lives. They helped me march forward, tailor my message, and believe that knowing about sensation can enrich everyday life. I am grateful to these men and women for the gift of their minds, hearts, and souls in my life and in the pages of this book: Teresa Brimacombe, Jessica Clark, Jane A. Cox, Brian Grubb, Chris Lewis, Daryl Mellard, Ellen Pope, Louann Rinner, and Linda R. Wilkerson. Other friends and family also shared this journey as well by nudging, listening, reflecting, and offering alternative viewpoints. They continually asked me how much progress I was making, and when they could get a copy of this book! I am grateful for their support as well: Carolyn Baum, Tana Brown, Beth Cada, Wendy Coster, Sally DeLozier, Jackie Dunn, Jessica Dunn, Jim Dunn, Susan Gardner, Mary Law, Charlie Lamento, Brenda Myles, Randy Netz, Becky Nicholson, Neil Salkind, Sara Salkind, Jean Sloan, Dave Smith, Phil Wassmer, and Tim Wilson.

Special note

There are many stories from people's lives in this book. The stories are not exact reports from individual life experiences; they are composites from stories people have told me about their life experiences as we have discussed the sensory codes, and how they play out in each person's life.

Learning about the Sensory Patterns

Section 1 gives you the tools to understand the sensory patterns. You will learn the basics about how your sensory systems work and what your reactions mean. Once you understand your sensory patterns and the sensory patterns of friends and family, you will open the door to an enriched life.

- Chapter 1 provides an overview about sensation, and why it is important to people's lives.

- Chapter 2 provides details about how each sensory system gives your brain information about your body and the world around you.

- Chapter 3 outlines how to crack the sensory code and understand your sensory patterns. You will learn the four sensory patterns that guide people's choices and decisions in life. This chapter also contains the first sensory Patterns Questionnaire, so you can get a general idea about your own sensory patterns.

1

Sensation Is Everywhere!

- Are you ticklish?

- Do you cut the tags out of your clothes?

- Do you need to jog hard to have a good day?

- Do you cringe at a sip of sour lemonade?

- Do you keep the shades down?

- Do you crave high volume on your ipod?

Your answers to these questions tell a lot about you. They provide a window to understanding how your sensory systems work, and when you understand your senses, life can be much more satisfying! There are several core ideas that guide our understanding about sensations and sensory patterns.

We are all sensory beings, yet our experiences are unique

If I ask you to describe a pleasant experience, you might talk about a sunny day at the beach, an inviting and comfortable room, or even an exchange between yourself and a loved one. As you told me the story, you would use lots of descriptive words to help me understand. You might use words like "warm" and "soft." Each of these words creates an image in both our minds because we have had "warm" and "soft" experiences of our own before. So as you tell me about the beach, you might say: "I love the damp, cool feeling of the sand on my skin." But as I listen to your story, I might think: "Hmmm, I don't think of the sandy beach as damp and cool; it's rough and scratchy to me."

I can see that the experience of lying on the sand is pleasant to you based on both your description and the inflection in your voice. And although I can appreciate your experience, I continue to be haunted by the itchy feeling that is coming over me thinking about sitting on the sand myself.

The words we use to describe our experiences reflect sensations. For example, the word "bright" involves visual input; "soft," "damp," "cool," and "scratchy" involve touch input. In fact, our sensory systems provide the palate for describing all the experiences we have.

> **We use sensory words to describe our experiences**

So everyone lives a sensational life. It's just that "sensational" means something different for each person. Some of us really like touch, while others would rather other people keep their distance. Some people are picky eaters, and other people will eat anything they can find. Even though people might not be aware of it, sounds, sights, touch, taste, smells, and movement affect us all day long.

Research has shown us that there are four basic ways that people respond to sensory experiences (see the Bibliography at the end of the book for details of the literature available). Imagine that there are four people being invited to taste a new and unusual food. Here is how they might respond:

"Mmmmmm!"

"Ach!!!!!"

"No thanks."

"What…oh, OK."

You have probably been with a group of friends or family when these different responses have occurred. The first person cannot wait to try something new. The second person hates the new food after trying it. The third person isn't even willing to try the food, and the fourth person misses the initial invitation and then goes ahead and tries it.

We experience life through our senses. We hear, taste, smell, touch, see, and move around. We have sensations inside ourselves that help us keep track of how our bodies are doing from moment to moment and day to day. We experience a sense of calm with some sensory experiences, and get overwhelmed with other sensory experiences. But just like the example of eating a new food, people will have their own personal lists of what sensory experiences are calming or overwhelming. Some of us readily search for new input, while others withdraw from situations to reduce the amount of input available.

The world is a sensory place

Sensation is everywhere. Not only are people sensory beings, the world is a sensory place as well. The world around us makes sounds, provides textures, offers tastes and smells, and contains a myriad things to see. We use sensory words to describe all of the physical characteristics of our homes, workplaces, parks, restaurants, stores, and any other setting. For example, a store might be described as bright, noisy, and crowded, reflecting the visual, auditory, and touch sensory systems.

We even describe objects with sensory words. Coffee cups are heavy (or light), smooth (or rough), brightly colored (or pale). Each of these ways describing the coffee cup reflects the work of our sensory systems to id tify certain aspects of the coffee cup. Sometimes it is easy to agree abou characteristics of objects, while at other times, people might differ i descriptions of particular objects. For example, when we describe "heavy," what rules have we applied to the cup? It is likely that we paring the weight of the cup to other cups we have held. So, if w held plastic cups, then nearly any coffee cup made of meta would be "heavy." However, if we have held many other ceran a coffee cup would have to be unusually dense to be called "l experiences (which are held in our memories) intersect world to help us decide how we will describe objects.

If anyone doubts the power of sensation, they onl marketplace. The marketing campaigns of prominen importance of tapping into people as sensory bein

- York Peppermint Patties has proclaimed "

- Pier 1 Imports has invited customers to "Get in touch with your senses."

- Hanes has launched a line of tagless underwear, a strategy to respond to people's experiences of scratchy tags; other companies have followed its lead.

- Kentucky Fried Chicken is "Finger lickin' good."

- The AT&T companies invite people to "Reach out and touch someone."

- Verizon asks "Can you hear me now?"

- The M&M company has drawn on people's experience with sensations by saying "Melts in your mouth, not in your hands."

- Miller beer has proclaimed "Tastes great, less filling."

With this book, you will know what the marketers have been taking advantage of all along—that sensory experiences affect people's decisions throughout each day. We are our sensations.

Sensation is the brain's source of information

The brain needs sensory information to operate. In fact, sensory information is the fuel that makes the brain work. So, to keep our brains active, we have to provide sensory input. Luckily, the world is full of sensory experiences, so it is not hard to keep sensory input flowing into the brain. The interesting thing is that each of us needs a different amount of sensory information to operate the best. Someone who needs more sensory information may show this by touching people when talking to them, or adding spice to foods; someone who needs less sensory information may show this by keeping their distance from other people, or by eating the same favorite foods each week. People develop individualized memories because of personal differences in needing and responding to sensory input. These memories enable people to understand their lives in a personal and unique way; the memories based on sensation.

The brain's source of information comes from the sensory systems

In this book, we will explore a unique way to understand yourself and others: through the senses. By paying more attention to personal preferences about sensory input, what those preferences mean, and how they affect your life planning, you can understand behavior better. With this understanding, you can make adjustments that will enhance your life satisfaction.

There are many ways to understand behavior and they are complementary to each other. Researchers who explain behavior in a cognitive or emotional way are informing us about those aspects of human potential. The research that helps us understand sensory responses in everyday life adds a dimension to understanding human behavior. Sensory responses work along with emotional and cognitive responses to enable people to know themselves better. The information in this book adds to our understanding; it doesn't substitute for other things we know about ourselves. It is just another helpful point of view.

2

How the Sensory Systems Work

The brain needs lots of information and that information comes from the senses. Sensory information helps us to understand our own bodies and the world around us. Our body senses let us know about the shape and position of our body and its parts, how our body feels when it is moving, and about the things we put in and around our mouths. Other sensations tell us about the world around us, including what we see, hear, and smell. Together, the senses help the brain create a map of your body and a map of your world; the brain uses these maps to figure out what to do each day.

Sensations that tell us about our bodies

The sensations that tell us about our bodies are strategically placed so that the brain knows about everything the body is doing. The touch sensors keep the brain informed about our skin; the body position sensors tell about our muscles, tendons, and joints; the movement sensors tell us about where the body is in space; and the oral sensors create a log of the characteristics of objects, food, and drink that go into our mouths.

Touch tells us about the edge of us

We associate touch with bonding and relationships so it is a very powerful sensory input. The touch receptors are in your skin. Some of them are close to the surface of your skin, and other receptors are deep in your skin.

Because the touch receptors are in your skin, they tell the brain where your edges are, thus creating a map of your body surfaces.

Touch receptors tell you
about the edge of your body

You get a lot of information from the touch receptors. A light touch on the skin, like the feeling of a feather stroking down your arm or loose clothing contacting the skin, is one kind of touch. Another type of touch is called *touch-pressure*, like the feeling you get from a deep massage or from firm, tight-fitting clothing.

As with all sensations, each of us has different reactions to touch. Some of us really like the light, tickly feeling on our skin, while others either shy away from this kind of touch, or even have a powerfully negative response such as asking the person to stop or pushing the person away who is touching us lightly. Light touch gives the brain an alerting message, "Pay attention!," so it is a useful sensation to increase the person's awareness of what is going on. Light touch can also be distracting or uncomfortable for some people.

Touch-pressure sensation occurs when you get firm touch on your skin. The most common touch-pressure experience is from tight-fitting clothing, like stretchy exercise clothing. This type of clothing presses against large skin surfaces, and therefore activates a lot of touch-pressure receptors in the skin. Touch-pressure gives the brain an organizing message, "Ah, there it is," so many people find comfort from touch-pressure input.

Position-sense keeps track of our body parts

Another important body sensation is our *position-sense*. These sensory receptors are in your muscles and tendons. When we move, we push and pull against the muscles, thus triggering the position-sense receptors. We can feel where our arms, legs, head, and body are even without seeing them because our position-sense receptors keep track of them from the tension in the muscles.

Some people are very aware of their position-sense receptors, and other people seem unaware of this sensory information. Athletes use their position-sense to refine their movements; they pay attention to how it feels inside their muscles and joints when they move. They can compare the feeling to the precision of their movement, and then make adjustments to the internal position-sense feeling to improve their movement patterns.

Position-sense receptors keep track of where body parts are in space

When people are less aware of their position-sense, it is difficult to make adjustments to movements. For example, this person would have trouble adjusting a yoga position based on verbal instructions. Repositioning a foot or leg based on verbal instructions requires the person to understand what "closer" or "rotate more" means inside the body. When people are less aware, physical, rather than verbal, repositioning can be helpful.

Position-sense receptors organize the internal picture of our bodies, and so are important for our ability to understand and adjust our body as we move and change positions. When you shift in your chair, you are not only maintaining your attention and circulation, you are also activating your position-sense receptors to keep your brain posted about where your body parts are. The brain needs continuous and current information about your body, so it can plan how to use the body to do things.

Movement sense monitors the body in space

Once you have touch to tell you about the edge of you, and position-sense to know where your body parts are, you also need to keep track of where your head is as you move. This is where the *movement sensors* come in. The movement sensors are in your head, near your ears, and they tell the brain all about how your head is moving.

Movement sensors keep track of where you are in space

The movement receptors can tell how fast and in which direction your head is moving. Some people love the feeling of head movements; they are the roller coaster riders and downhill skiers. Other people prefer to keep their movement receptors quieter; these are the people that want to ride the train that tours the amusement park.

When people get motion sickness, their movement receptors and eyes are not organized together very well. People who get motion sickness will say that they do better when they are driving or sitting in the front seat of the car; this is because they get better visual information when they can see what is going on. With additional input, it is easier to coordinate visual and movement sense input.

Oral sensations tell us about things in our mouths

Our mouth is a treasure chest of sensations. We feel textures and temperatures and we taste all ranges of sweet, sour, salt, and bitter. There are so many sensory receptors in our mouths that we can get a lot of information very quickly. Babies rely on their mouths to tell them about many objects, not just foods. Even adults chew on objects (e.g. pencils) other than food.

> Oral senses tell us about flavors,
> textures, and temperatures

There is no mystery about what people like and don't like in their mouths. All you have to do is mention a food, or even a flavor, and people will tell you how they feel about it. Some people will swoon over how good that food is, and may even describe their experience with adjectives like "creamy," or " crunchy," or "spicy." Other people will blink their eyes, make a face, or pull away; they will also use adjectives, for example, "sticky," "mushy," or "spicy," and a tone of voice that tells you the food is unpleasant for them.

Yes, people who like or don't like something in their mouths may use the exact same adjective, like "spicy!" Sometimes we can describe something to another person, and even agree about how to describe it, and still come to different conclusions: "I *love* how spicy that sauce is," or "I *hate* how spicy that sauce is." As individuals, we get to decide how we react to something, but these reactions are based on sensory information.

Oral sensations are unique because they are a combination of so many sensory experiences. We feel the texture of objects and food, we can detect the temperature by comparing it to our skin surfaces, and we can distinguish the tastes involved. And even though we can feel all these parts of an object or food in our mouths, our brains can also combine the parts and know that the object is a pear. Consider this quote from the movie *City of Angels*:

"I don't know what a pear tastes like to you…"

"…sweet, juicy, soft on your tongue, like sugary sand that melts in your mouth…"

The angel is asking the human being to explain her obviously pleasurable experience of the pear, and she uses words to describe the textures and tastes; taken together this is her experience of the pear. Now some of you probably don't like pears for some of the same reasons; perhaps the graininess feels unpleasant in your mouth, or you would say it is "mushy" instead of "soft." We each bring our own personal experiences to bear when we decide whether we like or dislike our oral sensory experiences.

Sensations that tell us about the world around us

Visual sensations map the space around us

Our eyes contain a huge number of sensory receptors that catalogue the light and color around us. As we use our eyes, we catalogue the size, shape, and color of the objects around us. As we build more and more memories of the visual world, our brains associate these images with words (e.g. ball, chair, dog) and make comparisons among the memories (e.g. that is bigger, this is brighter).

As our visual maps develop, we use those maps along with our body maps to figure out how to move around successfully. Each time we move, we also get new perspectives on the visual world (e.g. objects get bigger as we move towards them), which strengthen our memories.

Visual senses create a map of the world

People who are more sensitive to visual input will be bothered by brightness, high contrast, and unfamiliar patterns. These individuals will pull shades down, keep lights low in the room, and prefer monochromatic decoration. Other people will be delighted to have an excuse to look at something longer to find its interesting and unpredictable features (e.g. a piece of art), and will want bright, flooding light in the room and lots of contrast because these visual experiences are stimulating and pleasing.

Auditory sensations map the distance around us

Sound works in interesting ways. Sounds are all around us, and we figure out where sound is coming from by detecting which ear hears it the loudest. We can also describe the characteristics of sounds like we do with visual experiences. This time we talk about how loud the sound is and whether the sound is high (e.g. bird chirping) or low (e.g. rumble of thunder).

We build memories of object sounds and voices just as with the visual sensations. We recognize the sounds of our family members' voices and a friend's car. We frequently know who is calling on the phone by the sound of the person's voice. We can tell the difference between a metal and ceramic bowl when someone is stirring, and we can even tell if they are stirring with a wooden, rubber, or metal spoon.

Sound receptors map space and distance

As our sound memories collect, we begin to associate distance with sound. We can tell if a car is coming towards or away from us. We can make a good guess about how far away a construction site is by the way the machines sound. Sounds travel across distances, so we can associate distance with the sounds we hear.

It is usually easy to notice when someone is sensitive to sounds. They move away from noisy places, hold their ears, comment on the sounds, or ask for the sounds to be turned down (e.g. the radio, stereo, or TV). People who are sensitive may also notice sounds that others don't notice at all, like the sound of the motor on the refrigerator or the toilet flushing. People who are more comfortable with sounds, or who use sound to activate themselves, will use higher volume, or you may find them creating sounds with other objects (e.g. tapping the pencil on the table, clicking the tongue, rubbing a pad of paper along the furniture).

Smell sensations map the earth and other objects

Our sense of smell is a primitive sensory system; we detect the smell of objects and the world through our noses. A chemical reaction with odors enables the brain to categorize smells, and create a memory of them, as with all the other senses.

Smell senses are primal and connected to our emotions

Smell is closely linked to the emotional parts of our brains, and so sometimes smells can trigger emotions more quickly than other senses. Smell is also closely associated with the memory parts of our brains, which is why a smell can remind you of an event, a situation, or a whole scene from your earlier life. The smell of cinnamon and fresh bread baking might place you back in your grandmother's kitchen as a child, helping her to make breakfast for everyone. Cologne can remind you of a previous boyfriend; an industrial smell can place you in an old neighborhood. Smells activate complex memory patterns, so sometimes you can feel like you are reliving an experience from an aroma nearby.

As with oral sensations, people are very clear about what smells are desirable or undesirable. People's reactions can be very strong and distinct, leaving little to the imagination about how someone feels about a particular smell. The perfume industry counts on us having strong and positive reactions to someone wearing its products. Grocery stores and restaurants hope that the aromas from the produce and cooking will entice you to purchase more items. People might reseat themselves at a concert to get away from someone whose cologne or hair products are too strong to tolerate for the evening. Someone might avoid shopping in a store selling scented candles because the smells are too overwhelming. Smell is a primitive sensation and so we have very clear and distinct responses to this sensation.

Sensations affect behavior in everyday life

As you can see, sensation is part of everything we do. Our daily decisions about what to wear or eat, where to sit in a group, or how to complete our errands are related to the amount and types of sensory inputs we can manage. This may not have been part of your awareness until now, but now that you are considering the power of sensation in your everyday experiences, you will be able to make more informed decisions about how to harness sensation to your advantage no matter what you are doing.

Table 1 summarizes common reactions to sensory experiences. Check the table to decide if you are sensitive or enjoy each sensory input we have discussed in this chapter. In the next chapter we will explore your overall sensory patterns.

Table 1: Common responses in everyday life that reflect sensory systems

Challenging	Pleasant
You are bothered by touch if you: ○ are picky about clothing fabrics ○ want to stand away from others ○ don't want messy hands ○ cut tags out of your clothing	You enjoy touch if you: ○ touch people while talking to them ○ stroke clothing in the stores ○ fiddle with objects in your hands ○ get frequent massages ○ want pets and partners to have contact during rest
You are sensitive to body position input if you: ○ trip frequently ○ hold your head in your hands at the table	You enjoy body position input if you: ○ wrap your legs or arms around chairs ○ sit on your legs ○ use yoga as a primary exercise ○ use heavy blankets for rest
You are bothered by movement if you: ○ get dizzy easily ○ get car sick ○ stay away from rides at the park ○ avoid skiing or skydiving	You enjoy movement if you: ○ crave amusement park rides ○ love downhill skiing ○ select high-activity sports ○ have to get up a lot during work
You are bothered by mouth senses if you: ○ are a picky eater ○ aren't willing to try new foods ○ notice even small changes in recipes ○ have only certain menu items you order	You enjoy mouth senses if you: ○ chew on something continuously ○ are an adventurous eater ○ love certain types of input, like sucking from a straw, biting down on crunchy foods
You are bothered by visual senses if you: ○ keep the shades down ○ turn only a few lights on ○ prefer single tones in decorating ○ have sparse decorations	You enjoy visual senses if you: ○ seek lots of natural light ○ use bright lighting systems ○ have a collage of items on tables and walls ○ attend to placement of food on plates

Challenging	Pleasant
You are bothered by sounds if you:	You enjoy sounds if you:
○ wear earplugs to reduce sound	○ have music or TV on continuously
○ ask others to turn things down	○ sing, hum, or whistle
○ notice sounds down the hallway	○ make noises with objects
○ can describe a sound in great detail	
You are bothered by smells if you:	You enjoy smells if you:
○ move away from areas with scents	○ experiment with colognes
○ can smell food or gum on someone's breath	○ use smell to decide how cooking is working out
○ get nauseous while food is cooking	○ add aromas to the room
○ have to smell everything before eating	

Bystanders don't know what they are missing

Bystanders don't notice what other people notice all the time. Bystanders need more sensory information than others; things need to be louder, brighter, smellier, and faster for a Bystander to pay attention. Because Bystanders aren't aware of things going on around them, they are easy-going people. Bystanders can also seem unaware and oblivious to their surroundings, and family and friends can wonder if Bystanders are paying attention to them.

Bystanders are easy-going and can focus even in busy places

Bystanders need intense sensory input to notice what is going on. Increasing the intensity gives the brain more information. You can do this when you make objects weigh more, change an item's color or background color to make the item more noticeable on the table, or add a movement.

Bystanders miss sensory information all around them. They might miss sensory information that would be distracting to other people, which makes it easier for Bystanders to focus, and they might miss important sensory information, causing errors. Bystanders ask the same questions several times and may retrace their steps. Bystanders easily overlook sensory information that others find irritating, for example a person standing too close, high-pitched sounds, scratchy tags in clothing.

The great thing about being a Bystander is that situations aren't bothersome. Since Bystanders don't notice some of the sensory information, it takes a lot to create concern. Bystanders are also able to pay attention to projects because they are not distracted by sensory information around them. They won't notice people walking by, sounds from outside the window, or papers around the desk or table.

The challenging thing about being a Bystander is that sometimes needed information can be missed. The brain needs more intensity, and not every sensory experience in everyday life is intense enough. Bystanders will have to get into the habit of taking a lot of notes and checking in with others to make sure to have all the information you need.

Bystanders might also drive family, friends, and co-workers crazy because they don't notice things that other people expect them to. It is incorrect to assume that Bystanders are deliberately ignoring others; Bystanders are not noticing what is going on around them. People will have to call the Bystander's name several times to get their attention, and will have better success by including touch, or by getting into the Bystander's visual field.

You will recognize a Bystander because they:

○ are easy-going and easy to have around

○ are not bothered by disruptions

○ have to be called several times to get their attention

○ ask you to repeat things

○ get lost, or miss signs when trying to get somewhere

○ leave dirt on face or hands

○ have scrapes or bruises, and don't know where they came from

○ seem clumsy

○ don't comment on cooking aromas

○ have clothing twisted or crooked on the body

○ forget things in daily routine (e.g. keys).

If you have a Bystander in your life, you will have a pleasant experience. Bystanders are easy to have around; since they aren't bothered easily, family and friends have a lot of latitude in their behavior when around Bystanders. You can change the schedule of activities or the furniture placement and it won't matter to Bystanders. What can be frustrating is that Bystanders may miss information they need to notice. For example, as a parent, it is important to notice what the children are doing, and to give them feedback when needed; Bystanders may not notice children scuffling or bothering each other.

At work, Bystanders are focused on their projects, and are not distracted by things going on around them. Bystanders can also be oblivious to project details, and so need checklists or reminders to make sure all details are attended to. Bystanders do well in teams at work; they are easy-going because they don't notice things that might bother other people.

Bystanders are great companions on outings because they are not demanding about their needs. They can go with the flow, and will not be bothered by changes in the schedule or last-minute plans. Bystanders may need others to organize outings and provide some structure because

Bystanders may miss important details. Bystanders will be most plugged in during outings that have changes of pace throughout the day.

Avoiders want more of the same and nothing else

Avoiders love order and routine; things feel more comfortable when there is a plan. They don't like new sensory experiences so they try to get everything to be the same. When things change too quickly, then Avoiders get uncomfortable. Avoiders love to do things the same way every time. Routines provide comfort because the sensations are familiar to the brain; this familiarity keeps the brain from overreacting. When routines change, Avoiders might become anxious; changes mean new sensory information will occur.

> **Avoiders create routines to keep life peaceful and manageable**

Avoiders want to control the amount of sensory information they receive, and they don't want very much of it. Unlike Seekers who want more and more, Avoiders need very little sensory information to manage. Avoiders will look for time to be alone. Avoiders will shy away from social situations, especially situations that are less predictable. For example, a cocktail party is more random than a community meeting. They will rent movies for home rather than go out. Avoiders will pull the shades down, or even prefer the room without windows. They will prefer cooking at home or getting take-out, and will have favorite foods that they eat frequently.

Avoiders experience discomfort quickly, and to keep from feeling this discomfort, they withdraw or can become stubborn and controlling. We must recognize the discomfort Avoiders experience from too much sensory information at one time. For example, Avoiders may feel overwhelmed at the grocery store with the densely filled shelves and all the unpredictable sounds and movements; Avoiders might become irritable or aggressive because all the sensations in the grocery store are overwhelming. To manage grocery shopping, Avoiders might run into the grocery store for a few things at a time, or even have things delivered.

The great thing about being an Avoider is that life is orderly and peaceful. Avoiders' homes are a haven for them; rooms are sparsely decorated, and once they set up their furniture, it will stay that way. Workspaces are also tidy, and Avoiders put their work away each day. Avoiders have favorite pastimes and they stick with them; this makes them experts at their interests because they are so focused. Avoiders use the same stores and restaurants, so people know them in these locations. With the advent of the Internet for shopping, Avoiders can buy what they need without the sometimes over-whelming experience of being in stores.

The challenging thing about being an Avoider is that family and friends don't understand them. Avoiders are content to be alone, but others may think Avoiders are lonely. Being alone means less sensory information, and so Avoiders find this desirable. Being around other people can be over-whelming because other people are noisy, bump into you, have different smells, and are moving around all the time. When Avoiders live or work with other people, it is harder to control the amount of sensory information, and so Avoiders can seem rigid or cranky until they can regroup.

Avoiders might drive family, friends, and co-workers crazy because of their need to control everything around them. Avoiders want to reduce the amount of sensory information around them, and so may try to impose more order into situations than others want. For example, Avoiders might make rules at work that restrict other people's work, like insisting that all music and radios be turned off. Avoiders may create schedules for the family that make it more difficult to respond to last-minute opportunities, like an invi-tation to eat with friends at a later time than dinner is usually served.

You will recognize an Avoider because they:

- leave the room when a crowd starts to gather
- keep the shades down during the day and at night
- shop online, or shop at small neighborhood stores
- keep their workspaces clean and sparse
- use utensils and wash their hands a lot when cooking
- turn down invitations to large gatherings
- eat take-out or home-delivery food frequently
- have narrow food choices
- avoid escalators or elevators
- move away from people wearing cologne
- select solitary leisure activities.

If you have an Avoider in your life, be sure to find places the Avoider can go to get away from it all. Recognize that Avoiders need to have alone time to regroup, and are not rejecting you when they turn down an invitation to spend time with you. Take advantage of their ability to be orderly by letting them arrange storage areas at home and letting them do chores that are predictable, like cleaning the kitchen after meal time and cooking. Negotiate changes in routines ahead of time and provide ways for the Avoider family member to regroup before attending more chaotic social events, like parties.

At work, Avoiders are predictable and follow the rules. They can be counted on to meet deadlines and have materials filed in an orderly manner. Take advantage of the Avoider's need for order by assigning them scheduling, organizing, and structuring duties. Provide clear goals and expectations, and timelines for projects. If Avoiders cannot have separate workspaces, then identify strategies for Avoiders to get away from busy workspaces during the day.

It can be challenging to go on outings with Avoiders because outings also represent a flood of new sensory information. Planning the outings ahead of time can help a lot because it gives Avoiders time to consider how to control things that can be controlled. For example, you can pack favorite snacks and drinks so the Avoider doesn't have to deal with unpredictable foods or eating schedules. You can agree on the amount of time you will spend at the outing, to create a manageable time frame for dealing with the unfamiliar settings.

Sensors keep track of everything

Sensors notice most of the sensory information around them. Sensors will have very precise ideas about what is loud enough, bright enough, or soft enough. They will also comment on their perceptions about sensations to those around them. For example, Sensors will notice and comment about the volume of the TV, someone's cologne or may cut tags out of their clothing. Because they notice sensory information all around them, they can be very easily distracted as well.

Sensors notice what is going on, and have precise ideas about how to handle situations
. . . .

The great thing about being a Sensor is that they are very sensitive to what is going on around them. Sensors will be the first to detect a change in a person's mood or a circumstance, and so will be considered the most sensitive friend or family member. Sensors can be very creative because they notice more details than others do.

The challenging thing about being a Sensor is that they can easily be overwhelmed by all the sensory information. Sensors can hear things in the hall that others ignore; Sensors can be very picky eaters because they detect even small changes in textures, temperatures, and flavors in foods. Sensors may need to spend a lot of time managing their clothing, noise and music, food choices, and type of exercise to make sure that they get just the right kind of sensation from these activities.

Sensors might drive family, friends, and co-workers crazy with their need to have things precisely designed. Sensors can be vocal about what is bothering them, and this can feel like an imposition sometimes. Sensors are trying to get just the right amount of sensory information, and it is challenging to be this precise.

You will recognize a Sensor because they:

o are distracted by sounds

o have trouble working in noisy environments

o startle more easily than others

o are bothered by quickly changing images on TV

o have precise ideas about clothing textures

o pick the same foods at restaurants

o can describe the details of textures or flavors in their mouths

o get movement sickness

o select only a few rides at the amusement park

o prefer clean designs for the home.

If you have a Sensor in your life, cherish their sensitivity as a window into another way to see the world. Sensors notice things more easily than other people do, and so can be a great resource for making sure that details are being taken care of. Sensors can also seem overbearing because of their continuous commenting and feedback about the sensory events during the day.

At work, Sensors are very detail-oriented. Since they notice details, you can take advantage of this by giving them planning and tracking tasks in projects. Sensors will also need to have some control over their immediate workspace, because they need just the right amount of light and appropriate seating. It will be helpful to place Sensors out of office traffic areas to minimize extra movement and sound during work time.

It can be challenging to go on outings with Sensors because they need precision. They will want to be in charge of planning the details so that they have the best chance of getting the sensory information they will need during the outing. Sensors will need time frames for more chaotic activities, and will do better in more organized situations. Sensors will choose the same venues over and over again, because they can predict the type of sensory information they will receive.

What is your overall sensory pattern?

With this brief introduction to the sensory patterns, you are undoubtedly forming ideas about what your sensory patterns are, and may even be thinking about family, friends, and co-workers. It can be exciting to begin understanding behaviors that have been a mystery. Perhaps you have had an "aha" moment about a behavior that has been irritating or bothersome to you. When we see why someone might be doing something, it can be easier to give the person some slack.

The Sensory Patterns Questionnaire is provided at the end of this chapter. This questionnaire is an adaptation of the Adolescent/Adult Sensory Profile (Brown and Dunn 2002), which was used in the research to learn about sensory patterns in everyday life. There are also standardized measures for young children (Infant/Toddler Sensory Profile) (Dunn 2002), children (Sensory Profile) (Dunn 1999), and students in school (Sensory Profile School Companion) (Dunn 2006a). These measures are also used in professional practice by occupational therapists and other professionals. Information about these professional versions for research and practice is available at www.sensoryprofile.com. The Bibliography at the end of the book contains professional resources for readers who are interested in the background material.

Remember: human beings are complex! Even though we discuss each pattern as if you will be one type, this is not how people operate. When you look at the questionnaire, you will see that you will be somewhere from "this is *not* an overall influence" to "this has a *strong* influence" for each of the sensory patterns. Some people will have consistent patterns (e.g. a *mild* influence from all the patterns), while other people will have varying patterns (e.g. *mild* influence on some patterns, and *strong* influence on others). Every pattern is great because it reflects your responses, and when you know your patterns, you will be able to manage your daily life more successfully.

This questionnaire will give you a general picture of your reactions. You will see in the coming chapters that you will have different reactions in particular life situations because they present unique sensory challenges. For example, you may have mild responses at home because you have created a perfect setting for your own sensory needs; you may have stronger responses in public situations that are busier and noisier because your system is more stressed. It is the interaction of your sensory patterns and the characteristics of the life situation that tell the exact stories.

> You will learn that your sensory patterns are
> specific to every situation you encounter in life

You will also notice that you have a unique pattern of sensory responses within one sensory system. For example, Emily has many reactions to movement input:

> I love the feeling of sitting on a glider, rocking in a rocking chair, walking on a movable sidewalk at the airport, being pushed back into my chair as the plane takes off. However, I am also the person holding the bags and jackets at the entrance to amusement park rides. I observe that people seem to enjoy these experiences, but I find these movement sensations unpleasant. I like the feeling of riding on an escalator (the movement sensation), but I have to really concentrate on stepping onto the escalator because the visual movement of the steps makes it hard for me to coordinate my body to get on the escalator.

So, Emily prefers linear movement sensations (e.g. the moving sidewalk, the glider, the escalator), and doesn't like rotational movement sensations (e.g. going sideways and upside down on the roller coaster). We will explore these specific differences as you read about dressing, vacationing, and parenting; the more specific your understanding, the easier it is to adjust your life to meet your sensory needs.

In the following chapters, we will explore how sensory patterns affect specific parts of life. You may have stronger patterns related to your wardrobe because the touch sensations on your skin are very important to you, but once you have "comfortable" clothing on (i.e. clothing with *just right* sensations), you can handle other situations, like work or exercising. You may be more of a Seeker in your leisure, and more of a Bystander in your work setting. That is OK. You don't have to be in a single category. You just need to understand how sensory experiences affect your life, and this will enable you to make adjustments to make your life more sensational.

> You may be a Seeker in your leisure and a
> Bystander in your work setting. That is OK!

Give the questionnaire to a friend, co-worker, or family member to trigger a great discussion about behaviors that you notice about each other. In the following chapters, there will be more examples of behaviors specific to that situation (e.g. in relationships, as a parent, in your wardrobe) and lots of ideas for making adjustments to support everyone's sensory patterns in many everyday life situations.

A final note

As discussed earlier, looking at sensory patterns is only one way to understand behaviors and responses. With any behavior, there are several ways to explain its purpose and meaning; multiple explanations are complementary to each other and increase understanding because human behavior is complex. The discussions in this book are not meant to take the place of any other explanations of behavior. The information in this book is based on studies about sensory processing across the lifespan, and is meant to increase and expand knowledge about human behavior by offering an additional way to understand how people respond in everyday life.

Sensory Patterns Questionnaire

Read each item below. In the *white box* to the right of the item, write in the number that reflects how often you use that behavior in your everyday life.

Scoring key:

1: **Almost never:** when presented with the opportunity, you almost never respond in this manner, 5% or less of the time.

2: **Seldom:** when presented with the opportunity, you seldom respond in this manner, about 25% of the time.

3: **Occasionally:** when presented with the opportunity, you occasionally respond in this manner, about 50% of the time.

4: **Frequently:** when presented with the opportunity, you frequently respond in this manner, about 75% of the time.

5: **Almost always:** when presented with the opportunity, you almost always respond in this manner, about 95% or more of the time.

TASTE/SMELL PROCESSING	Seeker	Avoider	Sensor	Bystander
1. I leave or move to another section when I smell a strong odor in a store (for example, bath products, candles, perfumes)	█		█	█
2. I add spice to my food		█	█	█
3. I don't smell things that other people say they smell	█	█	█	
4. I enjoy being close to people who wear perfume or cologne		█	█	█
5. I only eat familiar foods	█		█	█
6. Many foods taste bland to me (in other words, food tastes plain or does not have a lot of flavor)	█	█	█	
7. I don't like strong-tasting mints or candies (for example, hot/cinnamon or sour candy)	█	█		█
8. I go over to fresh flowers when I see them		█	█	█
MOVEMENT PROCESSING	Seeker	Avoider	Sensor	Bystander
9. I'm afraid of heights	█		█	█
10. I enjoy how it feels to move about (for example, dancing, running)		█	█	█
11. I avoid elevators and/or escalators because I dislike the movement	█		█	█
12. I trip or bump into things	█	█	█	
13. I dislike the movement of riding in a car	█	█		█
14. I choose to engage in physical activities		█	█	█
15. I am unsure of footing when walking on stairs (for example, after bending over, getting up too fast)	█	█	█	
16. I become dizzy easily (for example, after bending over, getting up too fast)	█	█		█
VISUAL PROCESSING	Seeker	Avoider	Sensor	Bystander
17. I like to go to places that have bright lights and that are colorful		█	█	█
18. I keep the shades down during the day when I am at home	█		█	█
19. I like to wear colorful clothing		█	█	█

VISUAL PROCESSING	Seeker	Avoider	Sensor	Bystander
20. I become frustrated when trying to find something in a crowded drawer or messy room	▓	▓		▓
21. I miss the street, building, or room signs when trying to go somewhere new	▓	▓	▓	
22. I am bothered by unsteady or fast-moving visual images in movies or TV	▓	▓		▓
23. I don't notice when people come into the room	▓	▓	▓	
24. I choose to shop in smaller stores because I'm overwhelmed in large stores	▓		▓	▓
25. I become bothered when I see lots of movement around me (for example, at a busy mall, parade, carnival)	▓	▓		▓
26. I limit distractions when I am working (for example, I close the door, or turn off the TV)	▓		▓	▓

TOUCH PROCESSING	Seeker	Avoider	Sensor	Bystander
27. I dislike having my back rubbed	▓	▓		▓
28. I like how it feels to get my hair cut		▓	▓	▓
29. I avoid or wear gloves during activities that will make my hands messy	▓		▓	▓
30. I touch others when I'm talking (for example, I put my hand on their shoulder or shake their hands)		▓	▓	▓
31. I am bothered by the feeling in my mouth when I wake up	▓	▓		▓
32. I like to go barefoot		▓	▓	▓
33. I'm uncomfortable wearing certain fabrics (for example, wool, silk, corduroy, tags in clothes)	▓	▓		▓
34. I don't like particular food textures (for example, peaches with skin, applesauce, cottage cheese, chunky peanut butter)	▓	▓		▓
35. I move away when others get too close to me	▓		▓	▓
36. I don't seem to notice when my face or hands are dirty	▓	▓	▓	

TOUCH PROCESSING	Seeker	Avoider	Sensor	Bystander
37. I get scrapes or bruises but don't remember how I got them	▓	▓	▓	▓
38. I avoid standing in lines or standing close to other people because I don't like to get too close to others	▓		▓	▓
39. I don't seem to notice when someone touches my arm or back	▓	▓	▓	
ACTIVITY LEVEL	Seeker	Avoider	Sensor	Bystander
40. I work on two or more tasks at the same time		▓	▓	▓
41. It takes me more time than other people to wake up in the morning	▓	▓	▓	
42. I do things on the spur of the moment (in other words, I do things without making a plan ahead of time)		▓	▓	▓
43. I find time to get away from my busy life and spend time by myself	▓		▓	▓
44. I seem slower than others when trying to follow an activity or task	▓	▓	▓	
45. I don't get jokes as quickly as others	▓	▓	▓	
46. I stay away from crowds	▓		▓	▓
47. I find activities to perform in front of others (for example, music, sports, acting, public speaking, and answering questions in class)		▓	▓	▓
48. I find it hard to concentrate for the whole time when sitting in a long class or a meeting	▓	▓		▓
49. I avoid situations where unexpected things might happen (for example, going to unfamiliar places or being around people I don't know)	▓		▓	▓
AUDITORY PROCESSING	Seeker	Avoider	Sensor	Bystander
50. I hum, whistle, sing, or make other noises		▓	▓	▓
51. I startle easily at unexpected or loud noises (for example, vacuum cleaner, dog barking, telephone ringing)	▓	▓		▓
52. I have trouble following what people are saying when they talk fast or about unfamiliar topics	▓	▓	▓	

AUDITORY PROCESSING	Seeker	Avoider	Sensor	Bystander
53. I leave the room when others are watching TV, or I ask them to turn it down				
54. I am distracted if there is a lot of noise around				
55. I don't notice when my name is called				
56. I use strategies to drown out sound (for example, close the door, cover my ears, wear ear plugs)				
57. I stay away from noisy settings				
58. I like to attend events with a lots of music				
59. I have to ask people to repeat things				
60. I find it difficult to work with background noise (for example, fan, radio)				
TOTAL SCORE				

	Seeker	Avoider	Sensor	Bystander
Raw score				
This is *not* an overall influence on my behavior	15–42	15–26	15–25	15–23
This has a *mild* influence on my overall behavior	43–56	27–41	26–41	24–35
This has a *moderate* influence on my overall behavior	57–62	42–49	42–48	36–44
This has a *strong* influence on my overall behavior	63–75	50–75	49–75	45–75
If you have *moderate* or *strong* scores, mark the sensory systems you think affect this pattern — Auditory				
Visual				
Touch				
Movement				
Taste/smell				

Note: There are slight differences in the scoring for adolescents (11–18 years), and for adults 65 years and older. Please refer to Brown and Dunn (2002) and www.sensoryprofile.com to obtain this information.

Daily Life
and Relationships

In Section 2, you will explore how sensory patterns actually look in everyday life. Chapters 4, 5, and 6 crack the sensory code for the routines of everyday life, relationships, and parenting, respectively.

- Chapter 4 covers your morning routines, taking care of your home, going to work, and running errands. This chapter provides a foundation for discussing more specific aspects of everyday life addressed in Section 3.

- Chapter 5 looks at relationships. Whenever people have to negotiate their relationships with each other, different sensory patterns can collide or work in harmony with each other. You will learn how to make choices in relationships that meet everyone's sensory needs.

- Chapter 6 explores parenting. Children and their parents have individual sensory needs, and when parents can understand them, their interactions and management strategies with their children can be more successful and satisfying for everyone in the family.

After you finish Section 2, you will understand how to create a rhythm for your everyday life, which includes meeting everyone's sensory needs in the course of the day.

4

Sensational Daily Life: Living Each Day with Your Very Own Style

The routines of our everyday lives create an essential background for everything else we do. Because they occur every day (or every week, etc.), it is easy to overlook our routines, or to consider them unimportant. In fact, routines set a rhythm that affects all of our other experiences. Daily life involves managing our personal needs (e.g. hygiene, getting ready in the morning, bathing, communication strategies) and managing our lives within the world around us (e.g. running errands, keeping our spaces organized, managing money and time). When managing personal needs or our lives within the world goes awry, this can affect our work, home life, relationships, and even our recreation.

Opening story

Rise...and shine?

Andrea and Steve have been married for 20 years. One of the family stories that gets told over and over surrounds their morning routines. It has become legendary because the ways that Andrea and Steve tell the story don't even sound like the same event, even though they are living through the morning routine in the same space every day.

Here is Andrea's story:

Every morning I enter into consciousness with a jolt. My husband Steve has a completely obnoxious alarm, and even though we have lived in the same bedroom with the furniture and the doors in the same place, it seems that Steve has no memory of these arrangements. Nearly every morning he misjudges where the corner of the bed is, and bumps into it as he rounds the corner. So I am suddenly awakened; and I try to settle back down to at least rest a little more time, but it is not to be.

Steve's misjudgments continue…he bangs hygiene products onto the counter and into drawers. And even though I have asked him to close the bathroom door, he cannot seem to get the door closed all the way, so spears of light pierce across the room. And he insists on listening to the radio while he gets ready, which would be fine except that when he gets into the shower, he turns it way up so he can "hear it above the water pressure." For crying out loud, they repeat the same stories every half hour; it's not like he is going to miss anything.

We even moved his closet into the guest room so he would go elsewhere to get his clothing…great plan, but it hasn't worked out so well. Steve invariably forgets something from undressing the night before: his watch, a belt, so he comes back into the bedroom during his morning ritual. [sigh]

Steve says I am a crabby morning person (is it any wonder, with all these interruptions?), but the truth is that I am delightful when I am out of town by myself. I get up slowly and leisurely, introducing light and sound delicately as I move from sleep to awake. My colleagues at these meetings find me serene and pleasant in the morning. Steve says he doesn't know this person. I tell him he is exactly right!

See if you can find anything familiar in Steve's rendition:

I have a very special alarm clock. It took me many trials to find the one that I could count on to wake me. It makes this really interesting sound, not like anything natural, so I know for sure it is my alarm clock, and not something in nature. Before this alarm clock,

I would not arouse to the alarm going off, and my wife Andrea would have to shake me, or crawl over me to turn the alarm off. So I am so glad that I found this one, so I can wake up on my own.

When I get to the bathroom, I like to get myself charged up for the day, so I turn on all the lights and the radio. I make the shower really hot and I like to use the pulsing showerhead. I really like the exfoliating soaps (don't tell my guy friends!) because they give my skin a zing while I am showering.

I know that I have to get the same things done every morning, but I always seem to forget something, like getting a towel before I get into the shower, or remembering where I put my toothpaste the day before. I do spend time searching for something every morning. But I figure that this problem-solving gets my brain active for the day. Sometimes I forget things in the bedroom, and she gets so frustrated when I come in to get my belt, or my keys. What does she want me to do?

I love Andrea, but she is a downer in the morning. She picks at me over every little thing, and seems to get exasperated with me. I have suggested she get up when I get up, so that she isn't creating a conflict situation for herself, but she says she likes to get up more slowly in the morning. Although I cannot believe it, Andrea says that she is completely happy getting up when she is out of town. I think she just wants me to feel bad that I have to get up before her. She is always better later in the morning when I check in with her on our cell phones.

Andrea is a Sensor contending with her sensitivity to sounds, light, and movement in the room, and has a husband who is quite prolific at creating multiple sensory experiences as he gets ready. She wants to introduce sensory input slowly into her day; she needs to transition from sleeping and being awake. When getting up is perfect for Andrea, it would be hard to point to the moment between being asleep and being awake. Andrea continues:

There was a time that Steve also had a hard time getting up; he wouldn't hear the alarm go off. He feels proud that he found an alarm clock that does wake him up consistently. However, he is still groggy, stumbling around the bedroom and bathroom.

Steve is a Bystander, so he needs some powerful sensory input to wake himself up in the morning. He has to make the lights bright, the radio loud, the showerhead pulsate to get enough sensory input to get his system going. As we hear from the story, it has taken a long time for Steve to achieve routines that have the right amount of sensory input to have an effect on him, and he has had help. If he were a Seeker, he would have had lots of ideas about how to get up, and probably would be bouncing out of bed in the morning.

Andrea and Steve have some understanding about their different sensory needs. They put Steve's clothing in another room so Andrea wouldn't have to contend with Steve's "indecisiveness" about selecting clothing in the morning. They found a new alarm clock so Andrea wouldn't have to turn off Steve's alarm each morning. There are other strategies they might try. They could place towels on the counter in the bathroom so that it would still be quiet when Steve places hygiene products on the counter. They might want to place felt bumpers or change hardware for the drawers and doors in the bathroom. They could also put a self-closing hinge on the door between the bed and bathroom, so no matter what Steve does, the door will close. And if they add a footplate to the bottom of the door, very little light will get through. They could even change to a more solid door to reduce the sound that gets through.

Introduction

Daily life is filled with sensory opportunities. Sometimes these opportunities are helpful to our routines, and sometimes sensory opportunities interfere with a person's effectiveness. Getting just the right amount of every sensory input can be tricky. Small adjustments can make a big difference to how the day might go. Think of small adjustments you have made, and how they changed your day. Perhaps a particular toothbrush felt too firm in your mouth, and your mouth tingled all morning. Maybe a new detergent made your sheets feel weird, and so you didn't get good rest. When you tune into your senses, daily life is much smoother.

General considerations

Everyone's daily life routines are designed to meet the demands of that person's life. You have to think about what makes a really good day for you, and think about what makes a challenging day. You will find that sensory experiences are an integral part of what makes good and bad days. Andrea and Steve knew what made a good start to their days; they just had the challenge of how to get just the right amount of sensory input for each of them to get off to a good start.

Here are some general ideas about how people see daily life from each sensory pattern:

You are a Seeker in daily life if you:

o create a loud, bright space for getting ready in the morning

o squeeze errands into an already busy schedule

o initiate spontaneous conversations a lot

o use a lot of body language and gestures when talking

o change your house-cleaning strategies regularly

o find yourself "multitasking."

You are an Avoider in daily life if you:

o have serious brand loyalty for hygiene and cleaning products

o have set routines for getting ready, managing your day, and get upset when these routines are disrupted

o have a weekly plan for your outfits and repeat them weekly

o only shop when you must, and have selected stores that are the only ones you will use

o tend to have brief conversations, wanting to get to the point and retreat

o prefer e-mail and text messaging to talking on the phone or in person

o schedule meetings with agendas to reduce drop-ins.

You are a Sensor in daily life if you:

o like to awaken in a slow and leisurely manner

o are easily distracted by the activities of others around you

- struggle to keep your focus on your conversation when there are other things going on in proximity

- tend to tell others to tone down their music, talking, and other activities

- prefer early-bird times for dining

- like smaller boutique stores.

You are a Bystander in daily life if you:

- are easy-going about routines being interrupted

- leave the house without things you need

- have a hard time waking up in the morning

- lose keys, purse, or important papers in the house/office

- get home and realize you missed an errand on your list

- lose track of time

- receive feedback from family members that something is not cleaned up right after you have cleaned it

- tend to leave items piled around the house.

The daily life grid in Table 3 at the end of this chapter also shows you some simple comparisons across the sensory patterns.

Seekers in daily life

Seekers want more sensory input, and so their daily life routines will be packed with sensation. They will find ways to make even repetitive activities different from day to day or weekly because the changes introduce new sensory experiences. They will find alternative routes to work and may even take out-of-the-way roads just to see or hear or smell something new. Seekers will try new products, change the order of their morning or night-time routines, and create different organizing strategies for their bills and checkbooks.

Seekers are very active in their everyday life routines

Sometimes Seekers can get themselves into trouble in their daily life because of trying to meet their sensory-seeking needs. Routines are helpful because they are familiar; one part of the routine reminds us to start the next part of the routine. With familiar routines, we spend less energy figuring out what to do next and therefore can focus our efforts on other things. Seekers might miss something in their attempts to "seek" more sensory input. For example, a new organization for the bills might lead to overlooking a due date; an errand might be missed. So Seekers have to balance their need for new input with some reminder strategies so important routines don't fall through the cracks.

Ideas for Seekers in daily life

- Use scented and textured products in the bathroom.
- Arrange hygiene products in open counters/shelves to create visual interest.
- Place clothing in separate locations from each other to create more opportunities to move around.
- Install a variable-pulse showerhead to create choices of water pressure.
- Select highly textured towels.
- Run a set of errands together, and use different paths each time.
- Shop in larger stores and busy times.
- Use a videophone, camera phone.
- Create a checklist for completing home tasks so you don't get carried away and forget something.
- Use color-coded spreadsheets for your money management (e.g. for categories).

Bystanders in daily life

Bystanders are very easy-going about their daily life routines. They will have a basic plan for meeting their life-management responsibilities, but it will be loosely organized. They are not likely to have a set plan for errands or house cleaning, and will have variable times when they arrive home after work or other activities. Bystanders who understand that they need more sensory input to stay alert will have scented products for cleaning and bathing; they will make reminder charts for themselves and wear a timer watch so they can get buzzed when something needs to happen. Since they need more sensory input just like Seekers do (only the Seekers will be more focused on getting the input), many of the strategies that Seekers use will be helpful for Bystanders as well.

Bystanders are easy-going in everyday life

Bystanders can get lost in their everyday lives. They can easily miss cues that others notice (timer going off in the kitchen, lights going off in a store that is closing). They might repeatedly forget to stop for milk or cat food on the way home, and have to make extra trips out to patch over the "crisis" of not having the item when needed. Clutter can build up because the Bystander doesn't notice; the clutter becomes part of the decor of the room or office. Like Steve in our opening story, even daily routines don't ever seem to be *routine*, and therefore require more time and effort every day.

Ideas for Bystanders in daily life

o Make outlines in drawers and on counters showing where your hygiene products and equipment go so you will keep them organized each day.

o Select scented and textured hygiene and cleaning products.

o Move the location of clothing, shoes, and undergarments so you have to move around a lot to get dressed.

o Use a variable-pulse showerhead to provide more intense sensory input as you wake up.

o Use highly textured towels.

o Use a written schedule board to keep track of appointments.

o Use phone or PDA alarms to provide cues about time passing.

o Take notes during meetings.

o Use checks that automatically make a carbon copy.

Avoiders in daily life

Avoiders are very steadfast about their life-management strategies. They find strategies that minimize sensory input, and use them in the exact same way every single day because to deviate is to introduce unknown sensory input. Avoiders are minimalists even in tasks that must be repeated; they will place all their clothing into a very small space so they don't have to move around much to find everything for getting dressed. There will only be one way to keep the bills, and cleaning products will be in one bin that can be carried around. Avoiders will get up at the same time, leave and return at set times, eat at set times, and be very loyal to brands (because there are only a few acceptable characteristics, and when they find an item that meets that narrow set of needs, they want to be finished with searching). They will also have preferred stores and times for errands.

Avoiders are steady in their everyday lives

Avoiders become very disrupted by any changes in their life-management strategies. From a sensory point of view, changes in the schedule and plans represent uncharted sensory territory; just the idea that they will encounter unfamiliar sensations is overwhelming. So the best strategy is to control everything so there are no opportunities for sensory "assaults."

Ideas for Avoiders in daily life

○ Keep the lighting low when getting ready in the morning.

○ Allow extra time to get ready so you don't have to rush and become overwhelmed.

○ Use delivery services for groceries and other home products.

○ Keep a list when you run out of things.

○ Use gloves when house cleaning.

○ Design an exact plan for house maintenance/cleaning and go over key points with family so they know exactly what you need.

○ Plan outings ahead of time so you can be prepared for unexpected things that might happen.

○ Create a getaway space in your home so you can reduce the sensory input you have to contend with when overwhelmed.

- Create a signal so the family knows you are leaving to regroup rather than as an insult to them.

Sensors in daily life

Sensors are particular about daily life routines. Just like Avoiders, a little sensory input can go a long way for Sensors. They like order and rituals and are more likely to be vocal about their preferences than Avoiders (who will withdraw into their cocoon for safety). Sensors will also know what sensory experiences they do like, and make sure they get these as well because this helps them manage the rest of the sensory input that is difficult. For example, Sensors who like soft music because of its calming effect are likely to have the facilities to play soft music in the kitchen, bathroom, car, office, and even when exercising.

> Sensors are particular about their daily life routines

Sensors are very picky because their sensory needs are so precise. Even the best-planned life management rituals will get changed or interrupted, so Sensors can often become upset. People around them are too loud, air fresheners and other people's hygiene products are too strong, and lights are too harsh for their sensitive systems. Sensors create personal management plans to counteract the bothersome sensory input that is all around them.

Ideas for Sensors in daily life

- Create a specific place and routine for getting ready and stick with it every day.
- Plan your errands, and space them out during the week so you don't get overloaded.
- Shop during off-peak hours.
- Use unscented cleaning products.
- Draw the shades in your bedroom to reduce light in the room.
- When you find clothing that is comfortable, buy more than one of that item.
- Let your friends know your favorite places to eat/go out.

great strategy of moving to a different space that she can manage more successfully.

People give a clue about their sensory patterns when they talk about the types of stores they prefer. Large department and specialty stores can be invigorating for people who are seeking movement and visual input; they can be overwhelming for people who get enough visual input quickly. Small boutiques can be too confining for people who are sensitive to smells or touching, or can be comforting to people who need a defined amount of visual input.

A mother lamented about her son's birthday party:

> My son couldn't wait for his birthday party; he wanted to invite ten kids over for the afternoon. When everyone got there, it started being a little chaotic, which it certainly does with ten boys that are eight years old! He spent quite a bit of time with his hands over his ears while the other children played.

This boy couldn't handle all the sounds (and perhaps the movements too) that were going on (he is a Sensor for sounds). Mom knew having less children would have been better; I told the mom that she could also plan very organized activities to help manage the environment for her son, since he has a lot of friends.

Body products

There are many businesses and industries that market products for self-care and hygiene. These industries appeal to people with various sensory patterns by offering scented and unscented products, products with various textures (e.g. creamy, thick, granulated), products in color palettes, and even products that are to be used at different temperatures (e.g. warm wax treatment). By knowing your sensory patterns for personal hygiene, you can save both time and money getting just the right products for you without being swayed by a trendy product that does not meet your sensory needs. Go shopping for products with your sensory needs in mind so you get the most satisfying products possible.

Seekers are more likely to change their hygiene products periodically. They may change scents within a line, or may want to try a new line of products. They may also experiment with products rather than use them in the prescribed manner. Avoiders are more likely to find a brand and line of products and stick with them, and be annoyed if they are discontinued.

They may use fewer products as well. Sensors are also loyal to a precise regimen of routines and products, and are likely to have a lot of partially used products that were not "just right." They want "pure" products without heavy scents or weight on their skin. Bystanders may use whatever is around and available, and will take the recommendations of family and friends about what to use. They would likely profit from scented, textured, and colorful products (particularly to get them going in the morning).

A day in the life...

So with these introductions, let's visit a day in the life of a Seeker, Bystander, Avoider, and Sensor.

A day in the life of a Seeker

Xavier wakes up without an alarm. He is always eager to start the day (after all, there is only so much sensory input you can get while sleeping!). He turns on the TV to catch up on the news, and frequently flips channels while he is getting ready. Each morning he decides which of the showerhead settings he is going to use, and washes his body with a bar of soap that is encased in a natural sponge. He loves this sponge pouch for his soap because it gets his skin all roughed up and it makes him feel so clean and awake. He uses the highest setting on his electric toothbrush, and goes through a brush head nearly every month.

He always wears a thick form-fitting cotton t-shirt under his clothing because he likes the feeling against his skin. He found a brand that has some stretch to it, and they are his favorite.

Xavier is a handyman, and has recently begun to work on his own. He used to work for a construction company, and as they got bigger, Xavier's daily tasks got more repetitive. The boss called it "specialized," but it drove Xavier crazy to do the same thing multiple times a day. Now, as a handyman, he is a jack of all trades and gets to dig into many tasks in one day. Since Xavier is going to different homes, he travels by different routes every day:

> Another interesting thing that has happened to me with this new work is that I have to think ahead about how to get my errands done. I never know where in town I will be, so I am looking all around on my way to people's homes to see if there are any places I might use to pick up supplies, groceries, or get something repaired. I know a lot more about the

town now, and it's kind of a challenge to see if I can get an errand done on my way to another appointment, rather than having to make a separate trip for it.

Xavier has tried two ways of managing his schedule and his money thus far. The first strategy was very systematic, recommended by his banker, and Xavier found it tedious. Now he is trying a system that color codes the part of town the job is in, and although he has to look in each colored folder every time he reconciles his books, he feels more organized with this method: "I know I have covered all the bases when I have looked into each folder."

When he gets home, Xavier goes running with weights on his ankles and wrists and his MP3 player cranked up with pounding music. When he gets back home he turns on the TV in the living room and the radio in the kitchen while he makes dinner. When he sits down to eat, he split screens the TV so he can keep up with his favorite sports and police shows. At bedtime, he crawls into his flannel sheets and piles multiple blankets on top of himself.

Xavier has found many ways to make sure he gets intense amounts of sensory input throughout the day. He keeps a steady stream of sounds, textures, and changing visual scenes coming his way. He also gets a lot of input from the weight of his tools, and the pressure in his joints and muscles from running, squatting, climbing and carrying heavy objects in his work. He changed jobs from a position that was more repetitive to one that provides him with more variety throughout the day. Xavier has created a satisfying life-management routine that meets his sensory needs.

A day in the life of a Bystander

Rachel is a very contented sleeper. She falls asleep easily and doesn't usually wake up till morning. The phone ringing doesn't wake her, and she has had to get a flashing light attachment to her clock radio that she places under her pillow so she can wake up. She has put sheer curtains in her bedroom so the natural light can stream in as day breaks.

Rachel feels sluggish in the morning, and so she has changed her bedroom and bathroom areas around to help her get more energized:

The mornings were terrible, and I would always be running late because I would stop after every step; I would find myself staring off into space with one sock on. So I moved some of my clothing into the hall closet, put my sweaters in the back room, and keep my undergarments in a chest of drawers across the room from the bath. This way I have to keep moving around to get dressed. This has been really helpful, especially on days when I am indecisive about what to wear!

Rachel is absent-minded, and frequently forgets things she needs for the day. She has bought multiples of certain essential items so she doesn't have to remember to carry them from home to work. For example, she currently has four umbrellas. One is for the office, one is for the car, and one is for home. However, she had to buy the fourth one last week because she was running errands, and she had left the "car" umbrella in her office from the morning rain shower (it was sunny when she left work, so she didn't think about it).

Rachel has a cozy, cluttered living space. She tends to pile up her mail, magazines, and projects wherever she lands in her apartment, so she frequently has to move some things to sit down somewhere. The extra things around don't seem to bother her, and she just chuckles and moves things if someone brings it up.

She has set up direct withdrawal for paying her bills because the deadlines would pass without her attention; this has made things much easier for her money management. Her sister gave her a big write-on board for her kitchen wall, and Rachel writes meetings, events, and outings on it so she doesn't miss them. Her friends and family have got into the habit of calling to remind her of activities because they know Rachel might forget and feel bad for missing the event later. She is so fun-loving and easy-going that no one wants to miss times with Rachel.

As a Bystander, Rachel needs sensory input to be more intense before she will notice it. She doesn't wake up to the usual sounds and lights that wake the rest of us. She doesn't notice the piles developing around her home; they sort of become part of the landscape, rather than being detected as "foreign material." However, Rachel has figured out some strategies to help herself as well. She added vibration to her alarm system. She writes important dates on the wall so she encounters them every day. She moved her clothing around to increase the number of times she has to get up and move around while getting ready in the morning. These strategies help her get through her daily life without her sensory needs interfering; she needs more intense sensory input to keep her life management on course. She also set up direct bill pay, which doesn't provide more input, but rather automatizes a routine task; she doesn't have to remember at all now. She has created a combination of ways to keep daily life workable for her.

A day in the life of an Avoider

Omar is a very disciplined man. He takes pride in his highly organized home, schedule, and workplace. His bedroom is a cocoon; he installed quilted shades on the windows and encased them in a frame so that no light can leak in. He also installed soundproof panels to block out noises from outside the room. He wears snugly fitting long underwear to bed, sleeps on 500 count (higher-quality and soft) sheets and has a heavy quilt on top of the sheets. He tucks the top sheet into the sides and bottom of the bed, and carefully slips in so he is firmly tucked into the bed.

He awakens every morning at 6 a.m. sharp; he has turned his alarm clock volume to "0" because the jolt of a sound in the quiet room starts him off badly in the morning. He hears the click made by the alarm clock when it reaches 6 a.m. and this is enough to wake him up. He keeps the lights off in his bedroom; he has a light in the closet, so he uses this light to get ready. In the bathroom, he changed to a 20-watt bulb in the fixture so the light is minimal.

Omar is a very loyal customer. He has tried and thrown away many products so when he finds something that he can use he stocks up; he doesn't like it when companies discontinue his chosen products. The drawer in the bathroom has all his supplies and tools lined up so he can get cleaned up efficiently. He has several pairs of the same chinos, and wears them every day with soft, well "broken in" t-shirts.

Omar works as a computer analyst, and he has been delighted with a change in his company that allows him to telecommute. When he went into the office, he wore earplugs to dampen the sounds from the workers in the cubicles around him. The glare from the overhead lights drove him crazy and he swore he could hear them buzzing and see them flickering all day long. On really bad days, he wore a visor to reduce the glare into his eyes and onto his computer screen. Now that he can work from home, he has complete control over his workspace, and he gets a lot more done. He has no overhead lights, and he has selected a room without windows for his office to reduce outside noise that might bother him. He has one lamp in the corner, with a rheostat so he can tune in just the right amount of light when he needs it. Mostly he works from the light on the computer screen. He has many e-mail relationships for his work and prefers this type of communication over using the phone.

He has set a disciplined schedule, and he sticks to it every day. Omar exercises regularly to combat his sedentary work. He prefers to walk outside when others are at work, and he has some weights in the basement he uses. Omar likes to order his groceries and routine house supplies online, and has them delivered or shipped:

> Stores have too many things and people in them; and the stores move things around so I cannot count on them being in the same place from one visit to the next. I would just end up aggravated, and feel upset for a while after running errands like this. Now the things I need just show up! I love that. Sometimes my sister will get things for me too.

Omar has a simple weekly menu, and most weeks it remains the same. Sometimes, he will cook a large pot of soup and eat that all week long. He is not a big fan of spices or fancy sauces, and prefers simple plain foods.

He usually goes out on Friday nights with friends, and they have settled into a ritual of meeting in the same neighborhood place. This way Omar can order foods he knows, and doesn't have to contend with an unfamiliar place either. At home, Omar likes watching movies over and over again, so having cable has been a big boon for him.

Although others might consider Omar's life restrictive or dull, it is a very satisfying plan for Omar. He gets easily overwhelmed, so creating a life that is insulated from unfamiliar sensory experiences enables Omar to function better. A Seeker like Xavier would be very unproductive in Omar's world because there would not be enough sensory input to keep his system engaged. Conversely, Omar would struggle in Xavier's environment. Omar's choices demonstrate that he understands his own needs, and feels competent working and living within these parameters. In Chapter 5 you will see that Seekers and Avoiders can find common ground (after all, they both want and need to control what is around them) and forge a successful relationship by understanding each other's needs.

A day in the life of a Sensor

Gabby likes to sneak into her day on her own terms. She likes to wake up to soft music with a tiny bit of light spilling into her bedroom to let her know it is morning. She doesn't get right out of bed; she hits the snooze button several times before taking the getting up thing seriously. She loves this time to coax herself into wakefulness. When she gets up, she pads to the self-timed coffee pot to get some freshly brewed coffee.

Gabby has very clear ideas about her hygiene products. She was delighted by the product lines that all smell the same (soap, lotion, shampoo, powder), so she doesn't have to get a headache anymore from the clash of the product scents. It was hard to find the ones she could use, though, because the store had so many choices, and she could barely get to the checkout counter without being ill. She also selects smooth-surface soaps, like glycerin soaps; she likes to rub the bar right on her skin to get an even creamy feeling. Washcloths are too "tingly" for her.

Gabby is very proud of her dressing area:

> I found these tiny halogen lights that I can aim at the wall so the light isn't bearing down on me. Yet the halogen is such clear light that I can see the exact shades of my clothing. I like to have a crisp, clean look, and don't want shades to clash. My dressing area is a small walk-in closet, and it is so efficiently designed that I can stand in the middle and reach everything I need. I keep my wardrobe small; when there are too many things to choose from, I get flustered.

Gabby is careful about how many things she schedules each day. When her schedule gets too tight, she becomes edgy and snaps at others. She becomes less productive, which frustrates her more. She makes a "to do" list each week, and divides it into days, so things get spread out. For example, she spreads out her errands and does one or two each day; she knows that others try to do all their errands on one day, but she cannot imagine doing this. She writes everything in her planner, but then usually remembers anyway.

Gabby is very careful about not shopping during busy times. The noise, people bumping into her, random scents from products and people, and the continuous movement all around her is so distracting that she will forget what she came for, or will leave without getting her task completed. She also tries not to drive during rush hour because she feels that there are just too many things to pay attention to; she has to keep the radio off in the car anyway, so the extra challenge of traffic makes Gabby crazy. So she gets a ride or takes a cab.

Gabby's home is tidy, and although she likes to have friends over, she is a little tense during gatherings. She likes everything just so, and people just aren't as careful as she would like them to be. She can feel crumbs through her clothing when she sits on the couch later, and she notices every little thing that gets moved out of place. This is also why she has had to fire several housecleaners; it would take her just as long to get everything back in place after they cleaned for her.

Gabby is very sensitive to the sensory experiences around her. She has figured out which scents, colors, and sounds are pleasing for her, and incorporates them into her daily routines. She has identified high-risk situations (such as driving and shopping) and found ways to reduce her personal risk of overwhelming herself with sensory input. Yet she continues to interact with others, and go out into the world, rather than withdrawing into a cocoon like an Avoider would. Sensors get enough sensory input quickly, so they have to be mindful about the number and types of encounters during the day and week.

What about the weekends?

Our schedules change on the weekends. This change in the daily demands and routines also changes the sensory input that is available to each of us. For some people, the change of pace on the weekend is refreshing, and for others, the lack of structure can be a little unsettling. From a sensory processing perspective, how a person does is related to that person's ability to continue to manage their sensory processing needs along with the demands of daily life. With pressure to get errands completed, Seekers like Xavier might see an adventure before him, with lots of new sensory experiences available. Gabby might get flustered with too many errands to accomplish in a short amount of time; having a less productivity-oriented weekend might suit her needs better. With nothing scheduled, Omar might get too isolated, but he would want to select his activities carefully to make sure he didn't feel the need to retreat. Rachel might meander through her weekend, being satisfied to hang out, and yet be open to last-minute plans as well.

What about clothing, living spaces, work environments, and vacations?

Because these aspects of daily life have special considerations from a sensory point of view, there are specific chapters devoted to them in this book. At the end of the day, all situations and circumstances not only provide sensory experiences but are also affected by a person's sensory patterns. Understanding the impact of sensory input in every experience, and designing strategies to manage each situation, make life more satisfying.

And we are not alone

Our "day in the life" scenarios presumed that all our characters lived by themselves and could create exactly the life patterns they needed throughout the day. This doesn't happen to very many of us. More often, there are competing pressures in our lives, and we have to negotiate how to get our sensory needs met. Let's consider some changes and see what might happen.

What about parenting?

What if Xavier (Seeker), Rachel (Bystander), Omar (Avoider), and Gabby (Sensor) had two children to deal with every day? What would they have to do to get their needs met while parenting? Xavier might enjoy a playful getting up routine with his children, and might add in some rough and tumble play. Rachel might have play areas permanently set up in her home because the extra items in the space would not bother her. Omar might create a separate play room for the children, and have an intercom so he could check in on them. Gabby might have special storage bins for the children's materials so they would not clutter up the space. Chapter 6 provides lots more ideas about sensational parenting strategies.

What if they were partners to each other?

What if these individuals were each other's partners? Rachel's casual approach would be most challenging for Omar and Gabby, since they have low sensory thresholds, and would be overwhelmed easily by Rachel's easy-going style. For example, Rachel might leave piles of magazines and newspapers right where she read them; these piles would be immediately noticeable to Omar and Gabby, and would be bothersome to their need for order. Alternatively, Omar and Gabby's need for structure to manage their sensory needs might be helpful to Rachel (e.g. Gabby would keep everything in its place so Rachel could find things), and Rachel's easy-going approach might provide a spontaneous and safe outlet for Omar or Gabby (e.g. to try something new without being judged as clumsy).

Xavier might also be challenging for Omar and Gabby because of his high need to create more sensory input throughout the day; as partners, Xavier with Omar or Gabby would find separate activities to meet some of their needs, and plan certain specific activities together (e.g. a favorite TV show, a home-cooked meal).

There could be clashes even with Sensors and Avoiders. Although Omar and Gabby both need to manage the amount of sensory input they get throughout the day, they don't have precisely the same needs. Gabby likes to linger as she awakens, while Omar has a very precise timeline. Omar keeps visual input low with shades and low lighting, which might be a little too dark for Gabby. By discussing each person's specific needs (which Sensors and Avoiders can do since they are very aware of the details of sensory input they prefer or dislike), they could help each other with strategies to meet each other's exacting needs.

And although Xavier and Rachel both need more sensory input, the casual way that Rachel approaches life could be challenging for the more active approach that Xavier has to getting his needs met. Xavier could provide some of the extra input Rachel needs; for example, on outings, Xavier could point out the new route he had selected for the trip, and comment on the sights along the way. This strategy would give Rachel the extra sensory input (the talking, looking, smelling, hearing) she needs to stay focused.

Chapter 5 and other chapters can provide many more ideas for successful sensory negotiations to enhance the experiences of everyday life for everyone.

Summary

Daily life provides a great window into one's sensory patterns and how they look in activities. Each type of sensory processing has great features and challenges within everyday life. Knowing these factors can be extremely helpful to individuals and families.

Table 3: The daily life grid: comparisons among sensory patterns on selected daily life activities

	Seeker	Bystander	Avoider	Sensor
Morning routines	Arranges products in an eye-catching manner Bounces out of bed Completes multiple steps at once	Items are arranged haphazardly Hard to awaken Misses usual or key steps	Specific product brands in cabinet Gets ready in the dark Follows very clear routines	Small number of specific products that are organized on shelf/in cabinet Awakens slowly to soft music or radio Gets distracted during steps
Running errands	Lumps many errands into a "marathon"	Uses reminders from others to cue self	Uses online, delivery, drive-through, and drop-off services	Only a few at a time
Communication	Multiple topics running without difficulty Uses a lot of intonation and gestures	Needs to have comments repeated Misses intonation and gestures	Planned into day Short and to the point Tries for e-mail	Quiet settings Challenged by interruptions No or small gestures
Cleaning	Uses scented products Plays music or TV Random order and schedule	Items left out become the new background May miss areas that are obvious to others	Uses gloves Has a set schedule and plan Knows what "clean" is	Unscented products and uses small amounts Knows exactly where things belong
Time management	Free-flowing and changeable	Time is elusive; relies on external cues	Careful and organized	Precise and in small increments
Money management	Uses money to derive pleasure and make life interesting	Very relaxed approach; loses track of funds, but not worried about it	Balanced to the penny; the process is calming	Balanced is good, but process creates anxiety

5

Sensational Relationships

As human beings, we are drawn simultaneously to be individuals and to be connected with others. There are many reasons we are attracted to other people and an equal number of reasons other people bother us. Since the human experience is rooted in sensory experiences, relationships are also strongly driven by the effect of sensation on the partners in a relationship whether it is friends, lovers, room-mates, or co-workers.

Opening story

And we will be alone in our togetherness

Tom and Miranda would tell you they have a very satisfying relationship. Tom is an associate dean at a state college and Miranda is a radiologist at the regional medical center. Because of their positions, they both have any number of professional/social responsibilities throughout the year. Their colleagues rarely see them together, which most people find to be very odd since both Tom and Miranda speak fondly of each other when topics of partners come up. Most of their closest colleagues have also been to their home as well; they are gracious hosts, and create an intellectually stimulating environment for the evening.

When you ask Miranda about why Tom isn't at a particular event, there is always some scheduling conflict that prevents his attendance. In a conversation about the pattern of behavior, here is what Miranda said:

> It isn't that Tom doesn't like the people I work with; in fact some of them are our personal friends as well. He just doesn't do well in situations that are so unpredictable.

And here is what Tom says about his personal experience:

> It bothers me that people arrive in a haphazard fashion and seem to roam around the room randomly as if they don't know what they are doing. I can never tell who is coming toward me or some-one close by. I have to think "Do I know this person? Are they going to get into my personal space? Will they have some God-awful cologne on?" Sometimes all the smells of the food and people's hygiene products makes for a soup of nauseating propor-tions for my system. I can barely crawl out of these feelings to even be civil.

Tom uses very charged words here. Others might not use "haphazard" to describe people's arrivals and departures. Others might be delighted that people don't come all at once so they can greet each person properly. Some people won't particularly notice the coming and going.

Miranda's reasons for missing Tom's events are a little different:

> I am very picky about the texture of my clothing. This doesn't mat-ter in my work, where I can wear scrubs that I have treated with a special brand of softeners so they feel right. When I do have to go to meetings, I can keep one outfit available for this express pur-pose. However, at these events, women have certain "rules" about how we are supposed to look, and people notice whether you are wearing the same thing from event to event. It takes me a long time to find any clothing item in my wardrobe because it has to feel just right on me or I want to rip it off within five minutes of putting it on. I have left places, or got part of the way there and turned around because my shoes weren't right, or some seam was grating across my skin. It is just too much to contend with, so I hear about the events second-hand when Tom gets home.

But Tom and Miranda are happy to entertain together at home. In this context, they can control the amount of variability by planning the menu, the schedule of activities, the number of invitations, and when hosting in one's own home, Miranda has more ability to manage her wardrobe choices. They can have a pleasant evening attending to their guests, engaging in stimulating conversation, and relaxing.

Tom is an Avoider and Miranda is a Sensor. They both have low sensory thresholds and so they understand each other at a very primal level. Both of their systems get overloaded very quickly, so they have to manage their sensory resources carefully. At home by themselves, Tom and Miranda have carved out separate spaces for themselves and they have one common living area with the kitchen and living room. This way they can each retreat to a space they have designed for their exact needs without concern that someone will mess it up (remember, "mess it up" is relative to each person's sensory needs; we all have an idea of what is good and what is messed up based on what meets our own needs). In the living room they have created little spaces with the furniture, so they can be "together" in this room, and still have a way of partially retreating if needed.

Tom and Miranda understand and respect each other's sensory needs. They don't take any of the absences or retreats personally because each of them needs to get away sometimes. Others outside this relationship might be perplexed, but this plan works for them, and arguably keeps their relationship on solid ground.

Introduction

Quality relationships are built on sound knowledge about how sensory input affects both you and your relationship partner. People have to negotiate how everyone's needs will be met while trying to accomplish something (e.g. going out to dinner, working on a project together). In this chapter, we will focus on the ways you can negotiate your way to "sensational relationships."

By now, you are familiar with the basic characteristics of the four sensory patterns. Let's review very briefly how these general characteristics look within relationships; if you need more details, Section 1 of the book contains more depth for you.

Seekers in relationships

As you know, Seekers are good at generating new ideas and creating novel situations. This makes life interesting and sometimes unpredictable. Seekers think of alternatives when things are going badly, and can intensify situations that are already exciting and fun.

> Seekers generate new ideas
> and create novel situations

Seekers have challenges with keeping routines in place so that situations are predictable for others who might need more structure. Seekers like spontaneous planning and this can be difficult for others who are not Seekers.

Avoiders in relationships

Avoiders are good at creating schedules and routines. They like to be able to predict what will happen because familiar routines also provide familiar sensory experiences. They create calm, quiet, and orderly environments.

> Avoiders design schedules and routines

Avoiders have challenges with the unplanned things that happen in the course of the day. They are quickly overwhelmed by sensory information and so busy and unpredictable situations are too much for them.

Sensors in relationships

Sensors are good at noticing details, and so they are going to be more aware of moods, needs, and patterns of behavior. Sensors are also vocal about their own sensory perceptions, so there is no confusion about what their needs are.

> Sensors are most aware
> of moods and changes

Sensors have challenges with the busy sensory environments. Sensors can seem short-tempered because when they reach their own sensory limits, they will comment about it, for example, "Turn that down," "Don't sit so close to me," "Let's get this mess cleaned up." Because Sensors need to manage sensory input (they can only tolerate small amounts), they may create a lot of rules; we may discover the "rule" in retrospect when we have broken it unwittingly.

Bystanders in relationships

Bystanders are good at providing flexibility and an easy-going environment. Because it takes a lot of sensory input for a Bystander to notice a situation, they can let little things go by without bugging others about them.

Bystanders are flexible and easy-going

Bystanders have challenges with detecting situations that will require attention. Bystanders need a lot of sensory input themselves, and so potential danger might go unnoticed, or they might miss attempts to get their attention.

Negotiating sensational relationships

The trick to having sensational relationships is getting tuned into your own and the other person's sensory patterns and needs. Armed with this information, you can construct your experiences together so that they are very satisfying for both parties in the relationship. When we understand the sensory demands of our relationship partners, irritations become quirkiness, battlegrounds can turn into playgrounds, and differences in priorities become coping strategies.

Some sensory combinations can be more challenging than others, yet all combinations have the potential to be volatile or nurturing depending on how we can handle it. Think about Tom and Miranda; many could conclude that they have a difficult relationship because no one saw them together in public. Yet when we begin to understand the intricacies of their relationship, they actually have a very nurturing relationship. By understanding each others' sensory needs, they have been able to construct their personal and social lives together, both to get their needs met and meet their obligations. Tom needs to control the amount of input he receives, so staying out of busy social environments helps meet his needs. Miranda is very particular about what is acceptable for her, and so she has learned to craft situations that are satisfying within her limits. They also created home life so they can recharge with quiet spaces. If Tom or Miranda had partners who pressured them to go out more, this would create a sensory overload situation, and could lead to other tensions forming in the family.

So we have to get in touch with the sensory needs of our relationship partners to make sure we are meeting each other's needs. Any pattern can work as long as we give each other the sensory experiences we need.

Consider Ricardo and Samantha's friendship. They enjoy each other's company enormously. When one of them gets going on a story, the other joins in and embellishes as they go. They have a solid group of friends, and everyone loves being around both of them, but there are times that other friends bow out of activities when they don't have the energy to keep up with Ric and Sam's energy levels (they are both Seekers).

One of the things that Ric and Sam love to do together is cook. They cook meals for themselves and their immediate families, for formal dinner parties, and for large gatherings as well. They spend time just looking through cookbooks dreaming up their menus and making grocery lists. They usually spend a day preparing together. They "power shop" at the grocery store, scurrying down different aisles to gather needed ingredients.

They set out several recipes at one time and work their way through them, jumping from one to the other as they chop, stir, mix, broil, and brown things. This frenzy of activity is great fun for them, but occasionally leads to missteps; one time they burned the almonds they were trying to roast in the oven three times before they got a batch they could use. They kept getting distracted with other tasks, forgetting about the almonds until they smelled them charring.

Missteps occur with Seekers as they get overly excited in activities. This is an example of how seeking can interfere with a person's goals in their daily life.

There is one thing that Ric and Sam have to negotiate when they are working together. Sam loves to blast trendy, fast-paced music in the house so she can dance while cooking. The volume and pace of the music makes it hard for Ric to concentrate; he complains that he has to read the recipe over and over when the music is too loud. So sometimes Ric gets to pick the music and when Sam needs more input, she puts on her earphones and ipod while she works.

So, although they are both Seekers for most sensory input, Ric has some sensitivity for sounds and so has to manage sound in order to take advantage of his other sensory-seeking needs. Ric and Sam found a great compromise with the ipod as well; Sam can get her needs met without being disruptive to Ric. Best of all, Ric and Sam can load up on their sensory needs all day while cooking, so when their family members or friends join them for the meal, the setting can be less intense since the others are not all Seekers.

So every relationship requires some thoughtful attention and planning to take advantage of everyone's strengths. Without consideration of sensory patterns, relationship partners can get themselves into situations that become unproductive for everyone.

Imran and Carl are partners in a workgroup at the manufacturing plant. They have just received a project to work on that they are both excited about. They get the scope of work, timelines, and goals for the project from their regional manager, and are ready to begin their planning. At their initial meeting together, they share ideas with each other, select initial work tasks, and go back to their offices.

Carl begins to e-mail with Imran, and gets irritated that Imran is not responding promptly. Then Imran starts showing up at Carl's office to talk about the plans. Carl is cryptic during these impromptu meetings and becomes irritable over these interruptions. He e-mails Imran after each one to tell him his ideas. This pattern goes on for a few weeks, and begins to threaten the progress of their work. At their monthly division meeting, it becomes clear that they are not meeting their target timelines for the project. At the suggestion of the manager, they decide to meet face to face at a designated time.

Carl and Imran are very dedicated to the success of this project and have a good track record in this company, so they lay their cards on the table. Carl asks why Imran doesn't answer his e-mails efficiently (which by Carl's standards is within 30 minutes). Imran says he plans two periods during the day for responding to e-mail because if he does them all at once, he doesn't stay focused. Imran asks Carl why he is so cryptic when he stops by Carl's office, and then is quite articulate in his e-mails. Carl says random interruptions throw him off his concentration.

They work through the issues, and describe for each other what a good work plan is. Carl needs predictability to stay productive, while Imran needs variety to stay focused. They agree on a weekly 30-minute meeting to catch up. Imran agrees to make sure he has read all of Carl's e-mails by this time, and will bring any information that Carl has requested. Carl agrees to name his e-mails carefully so that Imran can see topics and organize accordingly. Carl has an alert for his e-mail, so if Imran wants to ask a question, he can e-mail with the tag line "I need something," thereby triggering Carl to respond without feeling interrupted by a visit. Imran sets up his e-mail so it will sort all of Carl's e-mails together each day so he won't miss them.

Certainly there are many reasons why co-workers might become unproductive like Carl and Imran. But for this conversation, let's consider that these workers' sensory patterns may contribute to this scenario. Carl is an Avoider at work, while Imran is a Bystander. They are both productive workers in general, but their lack of understanding about each other's sensory needs could sabotage their work productivity. Carl wants to be left alone in his office, and prefers e-mailing, which communicates without all the extra sensory input of face-to-face meetings. Imran is probably using the "get up and visit" strategy as a way to provide variety, which enables Imran to stay alert during the day.

Since they are committed to a successful project, they craft ways to meet both of their needs. Carl gets to limit his face-to-face contact; Imran gets time to process Carl's input via e-mails. Although they didn't come up with this strategy, it is sometimes also helpful for Bystanders to set their computers to alert them about incoming messages; this "interruption" can provide an alerting mechanism throughout the day. Imran seems to need more active input, like walking down the hall, which is why he was stopping by Carl's office frequently.

Some Avoiders might not like the pop-up alerts about messages, seeing them as distracting and overwhelming; these workers might restrict their e-mail time to one time per day. Carl is more bothered by sensory input that in-person contact creates (e.g. sound of voice, intonation, eye contact, the person moving around, the person's cologne), so the visual pop-up is not problematic for him.

As Carl and Imran continue with their project, they divide the work to take advantage of each person's needs. Imran takes all parts of the project requiring changing locations (picking up supplies, visiting the plant), while Carl takes on all the detailed drawings and documentation. In this way, Imran gets to move around, and Carl gets quiet focused time, and the project proceeds more smoothly.

Another important part of work relationships is recognizing that partners don't have to do half of every task to be equally contributing. By dividing the work as stated, Carl and Imran create a stronger work pattern; they are meeting their sensory needs, which makes it possible to be more productive.

The curious thing about relationships

We have been discussing knowing your own sensory needs and the needs of those around you throughout this book. However, there is another factor that plays an important role in meeting sensory needs and having satisfying human relationships. When another person is important to us, we can make some adjustments to keep the relationship satisfying. We may be willing to try something that we thought was unacceptable, and find a way to fit it into our lives because it is important to the person who is important to us.

Lindsay is in a new love relationship, and has never felt so happy. Lindsay is a Sensor, and this has created some challenges in previous relationships. She is particularly sensitive to touch, so negotiating her way into someone else's personal space and letting someone else into hers has been difficult. In previous relationships, the other person has felt rejected by Lindsay's negative reactions to their touches, creating distance. With Pat, she has been comfortable with talking about this, and they have found that asking before holding hands, touching each other's backs, and kissing helps to make it easier to be close.

When Lindsay and Pat began spending the night at each other's homes, more issues arose. Lindsay sleeps in a dark space with a very heavy quilt. Pat likes to have a fan because of getting hot during the night. Lindsay imagines that the fan will keep her up all night, since blowing from vents or open windows in the car is maddening to her. Pat is afraid of being up all night due to the heat of the quilt. The relationship is important, so they decide to try. They fold the quilt in half so Lindsay has even more weight, and is also protected from the air movement of the fan. Pat uses the sheet, and they place the fan so it blows on Pat's side of the room. Lindsay also sleeps closest to the bathroom so she doesn't have to walk through the fan movement if she gets up at night. Lindsay discovers that the fan doesn't bother her at all, and that the extra weight of the quilt makes it even easier to sleep.

In addition to our senses, we also have thinking brains, which enable us to reframe some things to accommodate particular situations. Lindsay will still be sensitive to touch, and will continue to manage this in her clothing, food options, and so on, but was willing to find a new way to sleep because of her decision to work on this relationship.

Negotiating intimacy in relationships

So, personal relationships also have intimacy and this involves sensory patterns and preferences as well. Getting one's sensory needs met during intimacy contributes to feelings of satisfaction.

Let's use touch as an example. We learned in Chapter 2 that light touch gives a "pay attention" message. For some people, light touch is exciting (e.g. this may be just what a Bystander needs), while for other people light touch input can be distracting to their ability to focus on their partner (e.g. being bothersome to a Sensor). Touch-pressure input (i.e. firm touch on the skin) is more organizing and can be calming, which can be a great tool for relaxing one's partner (which can be great for an Avoider), especially when light touch seems unpleasant for them. Seekers might also like touch-pressure because it provides such intense input to meet their sensory needs. People usually know what kind of touch they prefer. Sometimes talking about touch preferences can be an easier way to discuss intimacy; partners can show each other what kind of touch feels best separate from explicit sexual activity.

Other sensory inputs also contribute to satisfying intimacy in relationships. Think about what kind of lighting, scents, and sounds (including talking and music) are preferable. The following checklist might help get the conversation started.

What I really *like!* (✓)	Sensory input	What I don't *like* (✓)
	Light ticklish touch to excite me	
	Firm pressure touch to help me relax and pay attention	
	Light so I can see my partner	
	Darker space so I can concentrate on other senses	
	Scented room/products	
	Favorite scents	
	Soft music to calm me for focusing	
	Intense music to excite me	
	Talking to keep my attention	
	Quiet space so I can concentrate on other senses.	

Special considerations in relationships

People with different sensory patterns will encounter different issues within relationships. Knowing what might be easier or more difficult can guide our planning and negotiations with relationship partners.

Special considerations for Seekers

Seekers share the need for more sensory information with other Seekers and Bystanders so these relationships can be easier for the Seeker to manage. Seekers join in with their Seeker partners to create more activity, go along with changes in plans, or to do something out of the ordinary. Bystanders might not initiate new activities, but will be more active and responsive when the Seeker changes the schedule or keeps the day active. Seekers can follow their natural instincts when having relationships with other Seekers and Bystanders.

Seekers will have to be more attentive in relationships with Sensors and Avoiders. These people get filled up with sensory information very quickly, and so sensory input has to be controlled so they don't get overwhelmed. Seekers will have to make plans to get their extra sensory needs met when their Sensor and Avoider friends and family are not around. Exercising, active work settings, clubs, dining out, and community service activities can provide the means for Seekers to get their sensory needs met without being disruptive to Sensors and Avoiders. Schedules and predictability are the most helpful strategies for managing sensory input. Seeker family members can create a separate and quiet location for other family members to read or work at home. Seekers can create a signal with their Sensor and Avoider friends that indicates their need to get away; this is particularly helpful at large gatherings because these situations contain many unpredictable sensory experiences that can be overwhelming (just like with Tom and Miranda).

Special considerations for Avoiders

Because Avoiders need control over sensory input for themselves, they provide a great environment for Sensors and other Avoiders who also need controlled sensory environments. The natural structure for Avoiders keeps sensory input from being overwhelming. Avoiders will keep environmental stimuli to a minimum, for example, TV, stereo, or radio off or turned down so that the sound doesn't get distracting. They will have regular meals and dining choices, and a schedule for activities as well.

Avoiders will feel most challenged by Seekers and Bystanders. Bystanders need additional sensory input, and won't naturally get more sensory input from an Avoider. When Seeker friends or family members do things to get more sensory input for themselves, they can unwittingly overwhelm their Avoider partners. Seekers need to get their needs met away from their Avoider relationship partners. This can be in the basement, yard, or room with a door at home, or by doing things separately in social situations. During family activities like meal times, when everyone is together, the Seeker can be more active setting the table, serving, and so on, while the Avoider member can be seated at the table. Conversely, the Avoider family member might want to be away from a big table of people by staying in the kitchen until it is time to eat.

Avoiders and Bystanders face a different challenge. Bystanders need more sensory input to stay activated during the day, but they don't always create sensory input for themselves. Bystander friends and family can be very easy for Avoiders because they are not demanding from a sensory point of view. Avoiders can provide different seating with extra cushions, or give their Bystander friend jobs to stay active. Imran and Carl showed us how to negotiate a successful relationship at work by using their sensory knowledge to their benefit.

Special considerations for Sensors

Sensors may do best with other Sensors and Avoiders because they also have limits on how much sensory information they can manage at one time. However, Sensors are very particular, so if their "particular" issues don't match, other Sensors or Avoiders can also be challenging. Sensors have to take care that the limits they create are consistent with others' needs. For example, if an Avoider friend is most careful about textures in foods, the Sensor must include this consideration into cooking a meal, even if this isn't an area of sensitivity for the Sensor.

Sensors will be most challenged by Seekers in their lives. The spontaneity the Seeker displays can be unnerving for the Sensor. If not careful, Sensors can get into power struggles with Seekers because how each of them behaves to get their sensory needs met do not complement each other. The Sensor will want to maintain some control over situations because this also means controlling the amount of sensory input; the more the Sensor tries to control, the more the Seeker needs to introduce more sensory input, and the power struggle continues. Remember that each of you is trying to get your needs met, and needs just don't match. It is important for the Sensor to manage their time with Seekers; pick highly desirable activities so there is mutual motivation, and preset the time you will spend.

Ben and Sarah go to yoga together. At first they selected space right next to each other. After a few weeks, Sarah moved to the front corner of the space instead of the middle and back of the class:

> I love Ben, but he is so intense and active during yoga. He can't just do downward dog, he has to move his body parts to "loosen" them up during the pose. He is always adding something to the poses, which is so distracting to me. I support him to do his yoga practice however he needs to, but I needed to get in an area that would allow me to concentrate on my yoga practice too. The upper front corner reduces my distractions, and it improves our relationship after class because I am refreshed rather than tense. Isn't that what yoga is supposed to be about?

Ben is a Seeker and Sarah is a Sensor; they have found a way to create positive common ground.

Sensors create limits, and this can be somewhat helpful for Bystanders who might need some structure. The risk is that too many limits can reduce sensory input to levels that are too low for the Bystander to detect.

Special considerations for Bystanders

Bystanders will do best with Seekers because they create all kinds of sensory experiences for themselves. Bystanders will not be bothered by this high level of activity, and as a bonus, the additional input is likely to be helpful. They can stay engaged in the family or friend activities.

Jamie is much more likely to be on time for events when her husband Aaron is getting ready at the same time. Aaron is changing his mind about outfits, telling Jamie about something that happened at work, and continuously moving around the room. He also asks Jamie questions that keep her moving as well, for example, "What are you wearing tonight?," "Do you think I can get away with wearing my black loafers?" When Jamie is alone, she tends to be less directed, and doesn't know where the time goes.

Bystanders are also easy for Sensors and Avoiders to have around because Bystanders are less likely to create overly busy environments. However, the Bystander has to be careful that they don't miss what is going on; Sensor and Avoider relationship partners might not provide enough cues to support continuous interactions. Bystanders might also miss cues about the Sensor or Avoider's needs.

Bystanders are both compatible with and challenged by other Bystanders. Since both people are easy-going and not demanding, relationships flow smoothly overall. However, Bystanders need input, and don't create it for themselves, so Bystanders have to design reminder strategies to make sure they stay engaged or they will face some trouble.

Emil and Damien are room-mates. They are both easy-going which originally attracted them to each other when compared with other room-mate options. They didn't want the pressure of some of the other hall mates they knew. However, some things are slipping through the cracks. They have forgotten to get their meal orders in and therefore didn't have their packed lunches available when they went to the cafeteria. After missing two weeks of lunches, they made a neon sign on their door to remind them to get their food orders in. By having the noticeable sign on the door, other hall mates asked them about their meal order frequently as well, which increased their attentiveness to the task.

Planning sensational relationships

Human interactions are complex, and based on many things, not just sensory responses. However, when we understand this aspect of our experiences with each other, we are one step closer to feeling in charge of how things go when we are in relationships.

Remember each of us is in charge of ourselves. When we understand ourselves, we can make our own needs clear to our relationship partners. And when we understand sensation, we can also anticipate the needs of our relationship partners, multiplying our chances of successful experiences together.

The box below gives you some tips to get you started on your sensational relationships. I am sure you will have many more ideas yourselves after you start thinking this way.

Key: Match the relationship that may apply to you and your partner, friend, or family member. Each relationship has been given a number. Locate that number in the box below to find the tips to enhance your relationship.

Finding your match	Seekers	Bystanders	Avoiders	Sensors
Seekers	1	1	3	6
Bystanders	1	1	4	5
Avoiders	3	4	2	2
Sensors	6	5	2	2

Tips for sensational relationships

1. Ideas for relationships between Seekers and Bystanders
Remember

Seekers are good at generating new ideas and creating novel situations. This makes life interesting and sometimes unpredictable. Seekers think of alternatives when things are going badly, and can intensify situations that are already exciting and fun.

Bystanders are good at providing flexibility and an easy-going environment. Because it takes a lot of sensory input for a Bystander to notice a situation, they can let little things go by without bugging others about them. Bystanders need more sensory input just like Seekers.

Tips

- Make an outing out of running errands together; plan many stops to keep you activated throughout the errands.
- Change the locations where you visit and catch up on the day.
- If you have a "same time" event (e.g. happy hour), then change the place you meet, and if you have a favorite place, change the days and times you go there.
- Find longer routes to places you go together; change the path to routine places.
- Let the Seeker decorate; this will provide both of you with lots to look at, move around, and manage as you move through the home.
- Post a calendar with events for both of you (individually and together) so you can both refer back to it (the Seeker may over-schedule without this reminder, and the Bystander may miss important events).

- Select the far side of the bed for the Bystander; the extra navigating will keep awareness up for trips to the bathroom.
- Create "surprises" as part of your relationship.
- Talk about what you are doing as you do it.
- Hang sound-producing mobiles in the porch or garden.
- Use aroma devices in the house.
- Open windows to enable ambient sound to enter the home or workplace.
- Dance with and without music.
- Play TV or radio in background to get more environmental stimulation.

2. Ideas for relationships between Sensors and Avoiders
Remember

Avoiders are good at creating schedules and routines. They like to be able to predict what will happen because familiar routines also provide familiar sensory experiences. They create calm, quiet, and orderly environments.

Sensors are good at noticing details, and so they are going to be more aware of moods, needs, and patterns. Sensors are also vocal about their own sensory perceptions, increasing their partners' awareness of sensory experiences all around them.

Tips

- Use unscented soaps and lotions in your household.
- Create routines for everyday activities and stick with them.
- Plan ahead for changes in the daily routine or schedule.
- Create separate spaces for each other.
- Limit the time you spend in large gatherings and structure your time while there.
- Limit TV, radio, and stereo to one playing at a time.
- Keep windows and shades closed.
- Negotiate how and where you will spend time together ahead of time.

3. Ideas for relationships between Seekers and Avoiders
Remember

Both **Seekers** and **Avoiders** like to control their own sensory experiences.

Seekers need more input, so they like spontaneous planning and this can be difficult for Avoider partners. Seekers have challenges with keeping routines in place so that situations are predictable for their Avoider partners.

Avoiders like things to be predictable. Avoiders have challenges with the spontaneous things that happen in the course of the day. They are quickly overwhelmed by sensory information, so Seeker partners can be challenging.

Tips

- Post a schedule for daily routines and monthly events so that both of you know what is going on; this will help the Seeker to control overscheduling, and enable the Avoider to plan ahead for required activities.
- Create separate spaces in your living areas.
- Give the Avoider the opportunity to select a few public events to attend, and the Seeker to attend the rest of the events alone; this also gives the Avoider partner time alone which is desirable.
- Drive separately to events.
- Plan to have small groups of friends to your home.
- Use e-mail to communicate; this creates a record for both partners.
- Have the Seeker do the unusual errands.
- Have the Seeker partner use a Walkman, MP3, or ipod so the Avoider partner doesn't have to hear the extra sound.
- If possible, have separate bedrooms to allow each partner the opportunity to make the space a sensory match.

4. Ideas for relationships between Bystanders and Avoiders

Remember

Avoiders are quickly overwhelmed by sensory information, so they want to minimize the amount of sensory input available. Avoiders have challenges with the spontaneous things that happen in the course of the day.

Bystanders are challenged to detect attempts to get their attention, and so may be perceived as uncaring. An Avoider partner will limit the amount of contact because relationships could be overwhelming with sensory input.

Tips

- Post a schedule of activities; this will remind the Bystander, and allow the Avoider to plan ahead.
- Have the Bystander run the errands.
- Socialize at home with a few friends.
- Have the Bystander wear a Walkman, MP3, or ipod around the house or at work.
- Create a set menu for the week and post it in the kitchen so you can talk about it; this enables the Bystander to stay focused and the Avoider partner to predict what sensory input will occur.
- Let the Avoider make a list of what needs to be done to "clean up" spaces; the Bystander won't notice what needs to be done.
- Text message or e-mail with each other to negotiate activities.

5. Ideas for relationships between Sensors and Bystanders
Remember

Sensors need to manage sensory input (they can only tolerate small amounts); they may create a lot of rules. Sensors have challenges with the busy sensory environment that occurs in the normal course of their day. Sensors will comment about what is going on around them, for example, "Turn that down," "Don't sit so close to me," "Let's get this mess cleaned up."

Bystanders are challenged to detect attempts to get their attention, and so may be perceived as uncaring. A Sensor partner may become bossy as an attempt to control the sensory input in the situation; although Bystanders are likely to be easy-going about the bossiness, they may not recognize the meaning of the behavior as an attempt to control a certain kind of sensory input. By not recognizing the sensory needs reflected in the behavior, Bystanders may not anticipate this need in future situations, thus continuing the pattern.

Tips:

- Provide music background for the Bystander and let the Sensor partner decide what music and volume.
- Let the Sensor create the schedule of activities for the relationship.
- Create a set menu for the week and post it in the kitchen.
- Let the Sensor decorate the home, but be sure to place furniture in places that require negotiating spaces for the Bystander.
- Have the Bystander partner run errands, but the Sensor partner make the list.
- Have the Sensor partner drive, or be active in the navigating.

6. Ideas for relationships between Seekers and Sensors
Remember

Seekers need more input, so they like spontaneous planning and this can be difficult for their partners who need to limit input. Seekers have challenges with keeping routines in place so that situations are predictable for their relationship partners.

Sensors need to manage sensory input (they can only tolerate small amounts), so they may create a lot of rules for their relationships. Sensors have challenges with the busy sensory environments. Sensors can seem short-tempered because when they reach their own sensory limits, they will comment about it, for example, "Turn that down," "Don't sit so close to me," "Let's get this mess cleaned up."

Tips

- Post a schedule for daily routines and check off activities so you each know what to expect next.
- Add light and decorating sparsely to your shared spaces.
- Drive separately to public events so that you can each stay the right amount of time (Seeker longer, Sensor shorter).
- Play even-tempo background music to create a calm background.
- Let the Sensor partner select the routes to errands and outings.
- Fold bedding in half so each partner gets the textures they need and enjoy.
- Select favorite restaurants that provide variety on the menu; this way the Sensor will have predictability and the Seeker can experiment.

6

"Sense" Able Parenting: Negotiating Life with Your Children

In this chapter, we will consider the special relationships parents have with their children. Parent–child relationships are a special kind of interaction; knowing sensory patterns of children and their parents can assist in making these interactions more successful. This chapter outlines the skills and talents of children with each of the four sensory patterns, as well as the special challenges parents might face with these children.

Parents also have sensory needs, so the chapter also outlines the special skills and challenges parents face based on their own sensory patterns. The chapter also provides a discussion of each parent–child sensory pattern and how to negotiate that pattern successfully.

Opening story

Driving Miss Daisy

Vera has a lot of errands to run, and her daughter Daisy is making the trip harder than usual. Daisy learned a new song from her preschool program, and insists on singing it over and over again. Now that they are in the car, Daisy has added a "percussion" section to her performance, by banging on the car seat while she sings. Vera is having a hard time concentrating on her driving, yet she doesn't want to stifle Daisy's good mood.

When they get to the grocery store, Daisy reaches out for the produce, and almost falls out of the cart. Vera steers the cart too close to the shelving in the cereal aisle, and Daisy holds out her hand as they drive down the aisle: "Hey Mommy! The boxes are smooth, then they make a bump on my finger."

Vera, a Sensor, gets worn out by all the extra sensory input that Daisy provides. She recognizes that Daisy (a Seeker) is curious and somehow knows that her exploration is important to her development, yet she has a hard time with all this additional stimulation herself.

Vera abandons finishing her errands, and goes home so Daisy can play in a less confined space. At home, Vera can keep track of Daisy without having to hear every word and song she utters. Vera needs this regrouping time before she can make dinner. She will have to run her errands while Daisy is at preschool throughout the week.

As a Sensor, Vera will do better completing a small number of errands in short time frames whether Daisy is with her or not. By going home, Vera is being respectful of both her and Daisy's sensory needs.

Introduction

Being a parent is one of the most satisfying and challenging relationships of our lives. Parenting changes as children grow, mature, and develop their own lives as adults. Because of the importance of these relationships, it is helpful to have all the information possible to make them successful and satisfying for parent, child, and all family members.

Sensory knowledge can help parents understand their children's behaviors and their own reactions to their children. Sensory knowledge can also give parents more ideas about how to handle parenting situations. The goal is for both parent and child to get their needs met while guiding the child's development.

Parents have different strengths and challenges depending on their own style of sensory processing. The most important thing to remember is that by knowing your and your child's style, you can influence your family situation. When children and parents are getting their sensory needs met, life is much smoother as well.

Seeker parent

Seeker parents are good at generating new ideas and creating novel situations for their family. This makes life interesting and sometimes unpredictable. Seeker parents think of alternatives when things are going badly, and can intensify situations that are already exciting and fun.

> **Seeker parents are good at generating new ideas**

Seeker parents have challenges with keeping routines in place so that situations are predictable for other family members. Seeker parents need more input, so they like spontaneous planning and this can be difficult for other family members who are not Seekers.

> **Seeker parents have challenges with keeping routines in place**

Because Seeker parents share the need for more sensory information with Seeker and Bystander children, these parent–child relationships can be easier for the Seeker parent to manage. Seeker children are likely to join in with their Seeker parent to create more activity (e.g. rough-housing), go along with changes in plans, or to go to the Seeker parent to get permission to do something out of the ordinary. Bystander children might not initiate new activities, but will be more active and responsive when the Seeker parent changes the schedule or keeps the child active. With Seeker and Bystander children, Seeker parents can follow their natural instincts to meet their children's sensory needs.

Seeker parents will have to work more carefully with Sensor and Avoider children. These children get filled up with sensory information very quickly, and so sensory input has to be controlled for them so they don't get overwhelmed. Seeker parents naturally want more sensory input, so they will have to make plans to get their sensory needs met when their Sensor and Avoider children are not around. Exercising, active work settings, clubs, dining out, and community service activities can provide the means for Seeker parents to get their sensory needs met without being disruptive to Sensor and Avoider children.

Schedules and predictability are the most helpful strategies for managing sensory input for Sensor and Avoider children; Seeker parents can post the getting ready, dinner time and bedtime routines, and have the children mark off each part as they complete them. Seeker parents can create a separate and quiet location for these children to go to play or read, so the children don't have to contend with the hustle/bustle of family life. Seeker parents can create a signal with their Sensor and Avoider children that indicate their need to get away; this is particularly helpful at large family gatherings because these situations contain many unpredictable sensory experiences that can be overwhelming for these children. Seeker parents can limit the errands they run with these children. When it is necessary to run errands with Sensor and Avoider children, prepare them ahead of time; while on the errand, give the Sensor or Avoider child something to look for during the errand. By focusing the child's attention on the object of interest, the parent reduces the child's attention to the sensory experiences that are occurring around the child.

Later in the chapter you will read the story of Polly (a Seeker parent) and her children Todd and Victoria as they get ready for the day.

Avoider parent

Avoider parents are good at creating schedules and routines. They like to be able to predict what will happen because familiar routines also provide familiar sensory experiences. They create calm, quiet, and orderly environments.

> Avoider parents are good
> at creating schedules and routines

Avoider parents have challenges with the spontaneous things that happen in the course of the day. They are quickly overwhelmed by sensory information, and children are busy and unpredictable, thus creating a lot more sensory information than the Avoider parent feels comfortable with.

> **Avoider parents have challenges with the spontaneous things**

Because Avoider parents need control over sensory input for themselves, they provide a great environment for Sensor and Avoider children who also need controlled sensory environments. The structure that is natural for Avoider parents keeps sensory input managed so that these children are less likely to become overwhelmed. Avoider parents will keep the TV, stereo, or radio off, or turned down so that the sound doesn't get distracting. They will have a menu for family meals that contains simple food, and the food options will repeat regularly. Planning errands and outings ahead of time enables Avoider parents and Sensor and Avoider children to participate in these family activities. However, Avoider parents need to be sure that they control the sensory systems that their children need control over. For example, if the child is quickly overwhelmed by touch, the parent controlling sound will not be helpful.

Anna has a dream situation with her son Greg. Greg likes to have a very structured setting for his homework. The table has to be cleared off, and it has to be quiet. Anna likes quiet to work as well, so they work together after dinner. They have had to negotiate a few things. Greg wears earplugs when Anna is typing on her laptop because the clicking is distracting.

Since Anna and Greg are both Avoiders, and they want to avoid sounds and a busy visual work area, they are good study partners. It is not uncommon for two Avoiders to have to negotiate some things, though, because their tolerances may not match exactly.

Avoider parents will feel challenged the most by Seeker and Bystander children. These children need additional sensory input, and won't naturally get more sensory input from an Avoider parent. When Seeker children do things to get more sensory input for themselves, they can unwittingly overwhelm their Avoider parent. That is why it is very important for Avoider parents to provide an active play area away from the main living area for the Seeker child. This can be in the basement, yard, or room with a door that can be closed. The Seeker child can then get his or her sensory needs met without overwhelming the parent. During family activities like meal times, when everyone is together, the parent can give the Seeker child the jobs of setting the table, running into the kitchen to get food or more utensils, or another napkin. When driving in the car, it will help if the Seeker child has something to play with (not a noisy toy!) or something to look for along the way. Avoider parents can use their skills of providing structure to make it possible for their Seeker child to get extra sensory input in a more organized way.

With Bystander children, the Avoider parent faces a different challenge. These children need more sensory input to stay activated during the day, but they don't create sensory input for themselves. Bystander children can be very easy for Avoider parents because Bystander children are not demanding from a sensory point of view. The risk is that the Bystander children will remain unaware of many things that are going around them if parents and others don't provide extra stimulation for them. For Bystander children, Avoider parents can modify objects and situations to present the child with extra sensory input during activities. For example, the parent can put a squishy cushion on the Bystander child's chair for meals; the cushion provides a slightly moving surface, which encourages the child to make continuous small adjustments (small changes in posture activate muscles, joints, and movement sensory receptors) and so it is easier for the child to stay alert. Bystander children can wear earphones with music or a radio playing in their ears while doing chores around the house. Exfoliating soaps and net scrubbers in the bathtub can also provide additional input for the Bystander child during bathing. Storing clothing in inconvenient locations around the bedroom can provide the Bystander child with many opportunities to move about while getting ready in the morning.

Samina was in a great neighborhood for children, which she loved for her son Ashok. With many children close by, the children could gather outside or at each others' houses to play, and still have adults overseeing the activities. She had a difficult time when the children wanted to come into her home to play because the chaos of their movements, changes in activities, and the just plain randomness of their time together overwhelmed her. Ashok is a quiet child when alone, but seems to get all charged up with the highly active games, which included chasing, jumping, and crashing into objects and each other. These activities seemed good for Ashok, but she much preferred watching the children in the yard so she could stay a little distance from all the activity and still be available.

Samina was thrilled when she found a new service in her city. Fun City is an indoor play park for children. There are supervisors in every section, and parents sit in adjoining rooms where they can watch.

Samina is an Avoider, and her son Ashok is a Bystander. Ashok's low-key approach to everyday life is a good match for Samina, but also keeps Ashok from experiencing the type of play that other children enjoy. In the neighborhood, Ashok has lots of opportunities to get the extra stimulation he needs. Since all the activity is overwhelming for Samina, finding alternatives like playing outside or at Fun City are perfect options for them.

Sensor parent

Sensor parents are good at noticing details, and so they are going to be more aware of their children's moods, needs, and patterns. Sensor parents can also be vocal about their own sensory perceptions, increasing the family's awareness of sensory experiences all around them.

Sensor parents are good at noticing details

Sensor parents have challenges with the busy sensory environment that their children create in the normal course of their day. Sensor parents can seem short-tempered because when they reach their own sensory limits, they will comment about it, for example, "Turn that down," "Don't sit so close to me," "Let's get this mess cleaned up." Because Sensor parents need to manage sensory input (they can only tolerate small amounts), they may create a lot of rules for the family.

Sensor parents have challenges with the busy sensory environment in the normal day

Sensor parents do the best with Sensor and Avoider children who also have limits on how much sensory information they can manage at one time. Sensor parents like precision, and so they will insist on things happening a certain way, and may invent a lot of rules to live by within the family. Rules create boundaries and this can be very helpful to Sensor and Avoider children who also need limits. Sensor parents have to take care that the limits they create are consistent with the Sensor and Avoider children's needs. For example, if the Avoider child can only tolerate one type of socks or underwear, the Sensor parent needs to make sure that the rules about what looks OK for dressing includes these preferred clothing items. These children might also have limits related to contact with others as you can see with Nancy.

Graham sometimes gets exasperated with his daughter Nancy, even though he loves her dearly. They share their affinity for keeping living areas tidy; Graham likes to have everything inside cabinets and closets, and Nancy seems to love putting her toys away. Sometimes her desire to "pick up" her toys creates a challenge with making friends. She will only take one toy out at a time, so when a friend comes over to play, she might become upset when the other child takes another toy to play with. She complains that the other child "isn't playing right." Interactive play is difficult too: "They get too close to me and touch my body, and it feels prickly. I just want them to stay in their own place without touching me." When this happens, Nancy ends up playing alone again. Graham notices that Nancy seems content to play by herself. But he worries about her having friends.

Graham and Nancy are Sensors. They both like things to be orderly (this seems to be visual organization). However, Graham is worried that Nancy seems to reject friends with her very precise needs. She is sensitive to the touching that happens when children get close to her.

Parents like Graham can first acknowledge that Nancy seems content to be alone playing most of the time. It is the child's contentment that is a guide to what to do. However, Nancy will need to have some positive interactions with peers as she grows. So, Graham can structure play situations for Nancy, which take advantage of her bright awareness without triggering her sensitivities (in this case, visual and touch). For example, he can teach Nancy and her friends board games that are still organized visually, provide interaction, but keep the children in their own spaces around the table. This is a way to encourage friendships on terms that Nancy can manage well.

Sensor parents will be most challenged by Seeker children. The spontaneity the Seeker displays can be unnerving for the Sensor parent. If not careful, the Sensor parent can get into power struggles with Seeker children. Remember that each of you is trying to get your sensory needs met, and parent and child needs just don't match. It is important for the Sensor parent to create getaway places for the Seeker child so that the Seeker child can get the additional sensory input needed without being upsetting to the Sensor parent whose limits are reached very easily.

The rules that the Sensor parent creates can be somewhat helpful for the Bystander child who can be aimless without some structure. The risk with the Bystander child and the Sensor parent is that there will be too many limits placed on the sensory input available, and this limited input will not be sufficient for the Bystander child to get activated. Structured play schemas that are both predictable (good for the Sensor parent) and active (good for the Bystander child) are a good match here.

Bystander parent

Bystander parents are good at providing their children with flexibility and an easy-going environment. Because it takes a lot of sensory input for a Bystander parent to notice a situation, they can let little things go by without bugging the children about them.

Bystander parents are good at providing flexibility for their children

Bystander parents have challenges with detecting situations that will require parental attention. Bystander parents need a lot of sensory input themselves, and so cues that would indicate potential danger might go unnoticed. The Bystander parent might also miss their child's attempts to get attention, or to get their needs met. For example, a Sensor child may become bossy as an attempt to control the sensory input in the situation; although the Bystander parent is likely to be easy-going about the child's bossiness, this parent may not recognize the meaning of the behavior as an attempt to control a certain kind of sensory input. By not recognizing the sensory needs reflected in the behavior, the Bystander parent may not anticipate this need in future situations, so the cycle of behavior will continue.

Bystander parents have challenges with detecting situations that require attention

Bystander parents will do best with Seeker children because these children will be creating all kinds of sensory experiences that will benefit both parent and child. The Bystander parent will not be bothered by this high level of activity, and as a bonus, the additional input is likely to be helpful to the Bystander parent. When Bystander parents have higher activity around them, it is easier to stay engaged, so in this situation, parent and child could continue playing together more easily.

Harold and Mandy are married and now that they have a daughter (Bianca), their lives have become considerably more complicated. Issues that were barely noticeable, and could be considered "charming" before, have become bothersome (perhaps even irritating). Harold likes a lot of order, while Mandy is very casual in her style. Harold loves that Mandy is carefree and easy-going (he recognizes that he needs to "chill" sometimes, and Mandy helps him to do this). Mandy loves that Harold is so organized; she feels scattered and appreciates some of the structure that seems so effortless to Harold.

Now that Bianca is part of their family, the house has become more chaotic. Bianca is four years old and is an exuberant and spontaneous child. She has very free-form play, loves to create art, and might change outfits several times during the day. Harold gets increasingly agitated with Bianca's accumulating toys, supplies, and clothing, and cannot understand how Mandy seems unaware of all the clutter.

Harold (of course) made a plan. He decided that they would dedicate an hour every Saturday morning to tidying up the house. He and Mandy had to work on the plan for several weeks, because the first week, there were no specific rules. Mandy was satisfied, while Harold still saw *many* things still to be done. Mandy also insisted that they find a reasonable plan that was within Bianca's ability. They agreed that they would focus on the living areas (TV room, kitchen, dining area) since this was where the family spent time together.

Mandy got Harold to tell her exactly what was bothering him in each area so they would do what he needed (Bianca and Mandy had worked hard, and apparently were not cleaning the things Harold was bothered by). For example, Mandy and Bianca picked up toys from the corners of the dining area, but Harold was more bothered by art supplies on the table where he wanted to put the plates.

They made the Saturday morning clean up time fun. They took advantage of Bianca's energy to teach her about organizing her belongings. Mandy made a lower cabinet in the kitchen for Bianca's art supplies. Since Harold was fine with music, they "danced" their way through the morning (well, Bianca and Mandy did; Harold just hummed!).

As you can see, Harold is an Avoider for visual input (upset by the clutter), while Mandy is a Bystander (doesn't notice the clutter). They were able to negotiate their relationship successfully until Bianca swirled into their lives (a Seeker). Bianca is creating a lot of random visual input for the family, which is delightful for Bianca, provides input for Mandy, and overwhelms Harold. They have worked out a great plan for meeting everyone's needs. Harold gets more visual order; Mandy gets extra stimulation from moving around, dancing, bending, picking things up, and putting them away. Bianca gets to play as she needs to and then gets to learn organization while dancing and moving with her parents.

For Sensor and Avoider children, Bystander parents can be helpful in certain ways. These children need less sensory input to manage, and the Bystander parent is less likely to create busy or overwhelming situations for these children. Additionally, because they don't notice small things that happen, the Bystander parent is not critical of their child's need for really specific things. However, the Bystander parent may also miss opportunities to understand their Sensor or Avoider children's cues about what bothers them. By missing these cues, the Bystander parent misses chances to organize positive situations for the child in the future.

With Avoider children who have more of a tendency to withdraw when overwhelmed by sensory input, Bystander parents have to be careful that this child doesn't get ignored. Bystander parents have to create extra strategies to remind themselves to check on their Avoider children so they don't get disconnected from family interactions.

Bystander parents will be most compatible with and also challenged by Bystander children. Since both parent and child in this situation are easy-going, and not demanding, the family will flow smoothly overall. However, Bystander children need input, and don't create it for themselves, so Bystander parents have to design reminder strategies to make sure they provide their Bystander child with extra sensory input. The extra input will be helpful to both parent and child, so creating strategies that change the environment are the best ones. For example, having the stereo on with the "random" setting on the music can increase attention. Moving the toys and furniture around so there is more movement required to get to places in the home can also increase activity levels.

Donald loves watching sports. His pattern is to sink down into the oversized chair and stare at the TV for hours on end. His daughter Tanya loves watching with him; she turns off the lights to make it a dark room, with only the TV light, and she wraps herself in a cocoon with the blanket so only her face is visible. His son Brian also watches with his dad and either lies on the floor or snuggles in with dad. Donald and Brian sometimes miss a play, but Tanya always knows what happened.

Tanya is an Avoider; she loves the very low-intensity environment for watching the TV, and has wrapped herself up to create an extra layer of protection. Because she is so "protected," she can really pay attention to the games. Donald and Brian are Bystanders. The comfort of the room and low lights make it a little harder for them to keep alert enough to track all the plays.

Summary

The relationships among parents and their children require understanding of everyone's sensory needs. Tables 4 and 5 provide a summary of what to keep in mind for parents and children.

Table 4: General principles for the sensory patterns of parents

Sensory pattern of parent	Principles
Seeker parent	Seeker parents are good at generating new ideas and creating novel situations for their family. This makes life interesting and sometimes unpredictable. Seeker parents think of alternatives when things are going badly, and can intensify situations that are already exciting and fun.
	Seeker parents have challenges with keeping routines in place so that situations are predictable for other family members.
	Seeker parents need more input, so they like spontaneous planning and this can be difficult for other family members who are not Seekers.
Avoider parent	Avoider parents are good at creating schedules and routines. They like to be able to predict what will happen because familiar routines also provide familiar sensory experiences. They create calm, quiet, and orderly environments.
	Avoider parents have challenges with the spontaneous things that happen in the course of the day. They are quickly overwhelmed by sensory information, and children are busy and unpredictable, thus creating a lot more sensory information than the Avoider parent feels comfortable with.

Sensory pattern of parent	Principles
Sensor parent	Sensor parents are good at noticing details, and so they are going to be more aware of their children's moods, needs, and patterns. Sensor parents can also be vocal about their own sensory perceptions, increasing the family's awareness of sensory experiences all around them.
	Sensor parents have challenges with the busy sensory environment that their children create in the normal course of their day. Sensor parents can seem short-tempered because when they reach their own sensory limits, they will comment about it, for example, "Turn that down," "Don't sit so close to me," "Let's get this mess cleaned up." Because Sensor parents need to manage sensory input (they can only tolerate small amounts), they may create a lot of rules for the family.
Bystander parent	Bystander parents are good at providing their children with flexibility and an easy-going environment. Because it takes a lot of sensory input for a Bystander parent to notice a situation, they can let little things go by without bugging the children about them. Bystander parents need more sensory input just like Seeker and Bystander children.
	Bystander parents have challenges with detecting situations that will require parental attention. Bystander parents need a lot of sensory input themselves, and so cues that would indicate potential danger might go unnoticed. The Bystander parent might also miss their child's attempts to get attention, or to get their needs met.

Table 5: General principles for the sensory patterns of children

Sensory pattern of child	Principles
Seeker and Bystander children	These children need more sensory input throughout the day, so provide more opportunities for the children to charge up their senses (without overloading other family members).
Sensor and Avoider children	These children are quickly overwhelmed by sensory input, so work to manage sensory input for them (without making life too sparse for other family members).

Dealing with multiple children in the family

Many families have more than one child, and they frequently have different sensory needs. Navigating through this maze of differing needs can be overwhelming unless parents are perceptive about what their children's behaviors indicate, and have ideas about what to do in each situation.

Consider Polly's morning routine with her children Todd and Victoria. Polly awakens early so she can get some exercise in before she has to deal with her children. Exercising gives her the feeling that she can be calmer for the day; she likes to dance, walk briskly, or do some yoga. She watches TV news and uses her MP3 player for background music for the exercises. She uses a pulsing showerhead and rubs exfoliating soap onto her skin during the shower, which makes her feel invigorated as well.

She sets out to get her children going next; it will take several visits to get her son Todd to wake up and get ready, but she knows that her eight-year-old daughter Victoria will enter her daily rituals with habitual precision.

Todd is 11 years old, and is an easy-going kid. Polly has always been able to get errands completed and go to any type of outing with Todd. However, getting him up and out the door for any activities has been one of their biggest challenges. He seems to be in a deep sleep every morning, and moving from this deep sleep to awake seems like a trip up a very steep cliff. Polly has tried incentives, using things that Todd loves, but nothing seems to be enough to interest him in getting up. She has also tried making Todd go to bed earlier, but no matter how many hours he sleeps, Todd still struggles to awaken.

Polly's routine with Todd is to open his door, sing out his name, jostle him, wait for him to respond, and then turn on the lights as she moves on to Victoria's room. She stops back into Todd's room on her way back down the hall, and typically calls out to him several more times while she is getting ready. Finally, she makes him come out into the hall so she knows he is out of bed.

When Todd comes into the kitchen, he looks like he wrestled a bear in his room after getting ready. His clothing is twisted on his body, his shirt is buttoned unevenly, and he may have mismatched socks on. He is fine with whatever mom is serving for breakfast, and if she asks him to help to clean up, he pitches right in.

When Polly enters Victoria's room, it is like she has entered an alternate universe. About half the time Victoria is already awake, and she pops right up out of bed to greet her mother. Unlike Todd's bed, which is disheveled, Victoria's bed is crisp and tidy. In fact, Victoria is very specific about how she wants her bed to be, and fusses with it before bed each night. The sheets and blankets have to be tightly stretched across the bed, so that when Victoria gets in, it is like she is in a cocoon. She also insists on wearing her footie pajamas that she outgrew more than a year ago.

Polly and Victoria then proceed with their morning script, which they have perfected from daily practice. Polly has learned that any changes in the morning script will be met with resistance, and will start them on a dark and unproductive path. As long as Victoria has everything the way she expects it, things go smoothly.

For example, mom and Victoria make sure to lay out her toothbrush, paste, soap, and hairbrush on the bathroom counter every night so Victoria doesn't have to dig for them in the morning. They also select her clothing to make sure that they have everything that is acceptable to Victoria before morning. Victoria will only wear one brand of underpants and socks, and has only a few outfits that she will wear.

Since Victoria gets ready more quickly than her brother, she spends time with mom in the kitchen. She always has creamy yogurt and if mom wants her to have fruit, she has to blend it so it is smooth as well. Victoria will help make Todd's breakfast, but is not likely to eat what they make.

We can see that Polly is a Seeker parent who has two different children. Polly gets some of her own sensory needs met by getting up to exercise; she listens to music and watches TV at the same time. A regular showerhead is not enough; she has to use the pulsing head to get more input to her skin. She also uses a textured soap to add more zing to her skin. Others might find this routine assaulting, but Polly needs this intensity.

Todd is a Bystander, so he needs a lot of sensory input to support his daily activities. Polly's intermittent calls to Todd are not enough to keep him activated for getting ready in the morning. She can add some things to the morning routine to help Todd to awaken and stay awake while getting ready. She can open the shades to bring in natural light, or even leave them open at night so Todd begins to have natural light as day breaks. Although this would be bothersome to another person (like Victoria), Todd won't notice it right away. She can also turn on some fast-paced music, remove his blankets, and turn on an oscillating fan.

Victoria is a Sensor, so her sensory systems are loaded up quickly. She probably notices her mother coming down the hall, and this is enough to wake her. Her picky choices reflect Victoria's strategies for keeping sensory input within her narrow needs. She wants firm touch on her skin from her pajamas, the bedding, her socks, and underwear. When Victoria gets upset, it is because she is noticing sensations that are either unpleasant for her, or are unfamiliar. Sometimes this attention to details that mom sees as meaningless leads to some conflicts, but mom has learned to predict what Victoria needs, and mostly can provide a safe place for her.

Building your sensory parenting strategies

Every parent–child relationship is unique. One of the reasons these relationships are unique is because of the parent and child's sensory patterns. The box below matches parent patterns with child patterns, so you can get a head start building your pool of ideas that work for you and your child.

At the top of each section of the table, there is a reminder about what is easy or challenging for you as a parent, and what the focus needs to be for the particular type of child. Then each section contains a list of ideas to get you thinking about what your possibilities might be. Remember, not all the ideas will be applicable to your situation. If your child is not sensitive to sounds, then ideas about sounds won't matter. So read the lists, and select the items that are helpful to you and your family.

Key: Match the relationship that may apply to you and your child. Each relationship has been given a number. Locate that number in the box below to find the tips to enhance your relationship.

Finding your match	Seeker or Bystander children	Sensor or Avoider children
Seeker parents	1	2
Avoider parents	3	4
Sensor parents	5	6
Bystander parents	7	8

Tips for sensational relationships between parents and children

1. Ideas for Seeker parents who have Seeker or Bystander children
Remember

Seeker parents are good at generating new ideas and creating novel situations for their family. This makes life interesting and sometimes unpredictable. Seeker parents think of alternatives when things are going badly, and can intensify situations that are already exciting and fun.

Tips

- **Note: these children need more sensory input throughout the day so these ideas provide more opportunities for the children to charge up their senses.**
- Change the order of family routines so the child has more opportunities to be stimulated with new sensory experiences during the day.
- Store socks and underwear in different locations around the room so the child gets more opportunity to move around.
- Place items in distant spaces so the child moves around while dressing.
- Serve food on a contrasting colored plate so food shows up.
- Create "surprises" to keep the child's interest in these new sensory events.
- Use soaps with textures imbedded in them to increase sensation on the skin.
- Teach the child to use a loofah sponge or net instead of a washcloth to provide more sensory input to the skin.
- Use scented bath products to activate smell sensations.
- Incorporate sprayer into bath to vary water texture on the skin.

- Encourage barefoot play on a variety of surfaces (carpet, tile, wood, grass) to activate sensory input to the child's feet.
- Place favorite toys in harder-to-get places to increase climbing, crawling, and so on.
- Put posters/other pictures up at child's eye level to make the walls more interesting for the child.
- Provide toys that make sounds while playing with them so the child gets more input.
- Have child look for things as you shop or run errands to increase visual interest.
- Dance with and without music so the child gets more movement and sound input.

2. Ideas for Seeker parents who have Sensor or Avoider children
Remember

Seeker parents have challenges with keeping routines in place so that situations are predictable for other family members. Seeker parents need more input, so they like spontaneous planning and this can be difficult for other family members who are not Seekers.

Tips

- **Note: These children are quickly overwhelmed by sensory input so these ideas show how to manage sensory input for them.**
- Post a schedule for daily routines and check off activities with your child as you complete them so the child knows what to expect next.
- Create a play area with space away from other children to decrease sensory chaos during play.
- Press firmly on large surfaces of your child's body during bathing to provide calming sensory input to the child's skin.
- Let the child pick their own washcloth to find one that the child can tolerate on the skin.
- Find firm-fitting undershirts/underpants/panties to provide even pressure on the child's skin.
- Select undergarments with wide bands that fit evenly against the skin to decrease irritation that may come from thin elastic edges.
- Gather clothing for child to dress in one place to decrease the movement required during dressing.
- Select an assigned seat for meals to create a space the child is familiar with.
- Keep shades drawn and add light sparsely to reduce the light the child has to manage.

- Allow child to have one food at a time on the plate to minimize the conflict of colors, textures, and tastes.
- Limit large unstructured time in public to reduce the number of overwhelming sensory experiences the child has to handle.
- Use unscented products to clean toys to reduce the smell sensations for the child.
- Play even-tempo background music during play time to create a calm background.

3. Ideas for Avoider parents who have Seeker or Bystander children
Remember

Avoider parents have challenges with the spontaneous things that happen in the course of the day. They are quickly overwhelmed by sensory information, and children are busy and unpredictable, thus creating a lot more sensory information than the Avoider parent feels comfortable with.

Tips

- **Note: These children need more sensory input throughout the day so these ideas provide ways to charge these children's sensory systems without overloading the Avoider parents.**
- Place mirrors at floor level to provide opportunity for visual feedback about play.
- Include multiple foods in one meal to increase tastes and textures available.
- Change the order of the foods you feed the child regularly to continue to activate taste, touch, and smell sensations throughout the meal.
- Encourage barefoot play on carpet, tile, grass, and so on, to provide more touch sensations to the child's feet.
- Teach the child to sample foods on the plate to add variety to the meal.
- Provide extra lighting or colored lighting in play areas to increase visual interest.
- Get a Walkman, MP3, or ipod so the child can have extra sounds without bothering the parent.
- Select heavier objects for playing to increase sensory input to the muscles and joints.
- Practice a routine over and over to give the child more sensory input
- Paint one wall with chalkboard paint so the child has opportunities to touch the chalk and feel the texture of the wall when drawing on it.

4. Ideas for Avoider parents who have Sensor or Avoider children
Remember

Avoider parents are good at creating schedules and routines. They like to be able to predict what will happen because familiar routines also provide familiar sensory experiences. They create calm, quiet, and orderly environments.

Tips

- **Note: These children are quickly overwhelmed by sensory input so these ideas show how to manage sensory input for them.**
- Get rid of undergarments (diapers, panties, socks) that have distinct elastic bands on them; children will feel like the bands are cutting into them.
- Provide a predictable set of foods for meal times so the child can eat with the family without being overwhelmed by unfamiliar textures, tastes, and smells.
- Use unscented soaps and lotions for bathing to reduce the smells for the child.
- Create routines for everyday activities and stick with them so the child has less unfamiliar sensory information to deal with.
- When you need to change the routines, tell the child ahead of time so the child is less surprised by new sensory inputs when the time comes.
- Keep shades drawn in rooms, add light sparsely so the child is not overwhelmed with visual sensory input.
- Use properly sized seats/chairs with foam cushions; this will provide even, firm touch to the skin.
- Have seating available, so young children don't have to be held all the time; holding children provides continuously changing input to the skin, and may be overwhelming.
- Keep additives out of clothing (such as starch) to reduce the sensory input from the clothing to the skin.
- Use unscented laundry products so the child's clothing doesn't have any extra smells.
- Notice where vents blow in your home, and direct them away from the child's seating or play areas to reduce the breeze on the child's skin.
- Limit the time you spend in large family gatherings because these situations are full of unpredictable sensory experiences that can overwhelm the child.
- Limit TV, radio, and stereo to one playing at a time in the home so the child does not have to contend with competing sounds.
- Close windows to reduce external sounds for the child.

- Provide a quiet out-of-the-way place for the child to calm down when upset by too much sensory input.
- Select tight, firm-fitting clothing with some stretch in it; the firm feeling on the skin can be calming for the child.
- Remove loose-fitting clothing from the child's wardrobe unless the child can wear tight-fitting clothing underneath (e.g. bike pants, dance leotards).
- Place plain sheets over toy shelves to reduce visual distractions.
- Carry foam earplugs with you (for the child) in case you end up in a noisy place.
- Select chores for the child that involve pushing, pulling, or carrying heavy objects (e.g. bringing groceries into the home, taking out trash bins, mowing the lawn with a push mower, vacuuming); these activities provide calming sensory input for the child.

5. Ideas for Sensor parents who have Seeker or Bystander children

Remember

Sensor parents have challenges with the busy sensory environment that their children create in the normal course of their day. Sensor parents can seem short-tempered because when they reach their own sensory limits, they will comment about it, for example, "Turn that down," "Don't sit so close to me," "Let's get this mess cleaned up." Because Sensor parents need to manage sensory input (they can only tolerate small amounts), they may create a lot of rules for the family.

Tips

- **Note: These children need more sensory input throughout the day so these ideas show how to do this without making it difficult for the Sensor parents.**
- Be extra aware of safety measures for this child, who may not notice objects, stairs, or changes in terrain, and add sensory cues for the child (e.g. add colored tape to edges of stairs).
- Add texture to handles and other toy surfaces so the child gets more touch input.
- Provide background music that you like to increase auditory input for the child.
- Place desirable toys in hard-to-get places to increase climbing, crawling, and so on.
- Select highly textured, bright-colored clothing so the child has more touch and visual input from dressing.
- Teach the child to use a netting scrubber in the tub to increase sensation to the skin.

6. Ideas for Sensor parents who have Sensor or Avoider children

Remember

Sensor parents are good at noticing details, and so they are going to be more aware of their children's moods, needs, and patterns. Sensor parents can also be vocal about their own sensory perceptions, increasing the family's awareness of sensory experiences all around them.

Tips

- **Note: these children are quickly overwhelmed by sensory input so these ideas show how to manage sensory input for them.**
- Be particular about temperature of foods you serve; closer to room temperature may be best.
- Find ways for your child to play quietly and with little movement to reduce body sensations.
- Plan toy set-ups so the child can reach for things more easily to minimize extra movement and body sensation input while playing.
- Notice which kinds of light your child likes/dislikes (e.g. fluorescent, halogen) so you provide the visual input that the child can manage best.
- Notice clothing your child likes and stick with these fabrics and textures so the child doesn't have to contend with unfamiliar sensations on the skin.
- Direct fans away from the child, so they don't blow on the skin.
- Structure the time at family gatherings so the child can predict what will happen in this unpredictable sensory environment.
- Organize alone time for the child, recognizing that this child needs less sensory input to regroup.
- Find closed-in quiet places for the child to play/rest (they have less sensory features), such as a room with less windows.
- Identify flavors, scents, and textures your child likes and use them exclusively in the home so that daily routines are not disrupted with unfamiliar sensory input.
- Wrap young children tightly in their blankets because firm touching provides calming input to the skin.
- Construct activities in smaller parts and prepare the child for each one ahead of time to reduce the chances for surprise sensory experiences.
- Create small, tight spaces for this child to play, read, and so on (e.g. small tent in the basement, a fort in the yard) so the sensory environment is more manageable.

7. Ideas for Bystander parents who have Seeker or Bystander children

Remember

Bystander parents are good at providing their children with flexibility and an easy-going environment. Because it takes a lot of sensory input for a Bystander parent to notice a situation, they can let little things go by without bugging the children about them. Bystander parents need more sensory input just like Seeker and Bystander children.

Tips

- **Note: These children need more sensory input throughout the day so these ideas show how to charge the children's sensory systems.**
- Add new textures, temperatures, aromas, tastes to foods during meal time to increase sensory experiences.
- Talk about what the child/you are doing as you do it to increase auditory experiences to the routines.
- Provide toys that make sounds/move/change while playing with them so the child gets additional input while playing.
- Use aroma devices in the house to increase smell input in places the child frequents.
- Rough-house with the child to provide yourself and the child with additional body sensations.
- Put toys away one at a time in a distant toy box to increase movement opportunities.
- Put posters/other pictures up at the child's eye level to increase visual interest for the child.
- Hum/sing to songs, make up rhymes, add movements while playing to intensify sensory experiences for the child.
- Open windows to enable ambient sound to enter and activate the child's sensory interest in the larger environment.
- Get a mini trampoline so the child can jump on their own in a specified location.
- Use scented soaps during bath and changing times to add touch and scents to these daily routines.
- Find longer routes to tasks (e.g. longer paths to table, obstacle courses in play areas) so the child has more body and movement input.
- Dance with and without music to add body, auditory, and movement sensations.
- Garden/dig in the dirt/sand so the child can get more body, touch, smell, and visual sensations.
- Finger paint, and add textures to the paint so the child gets more feedback from the hands while painting.

○ Use lotions/soaps and creams with texture/scents to intensify sensory input for the child.

○ Play TV or radio in background so the child gets more environmental stimulation.

8. Ideas for Bystander parents who have Sensor or Avoider children
Remember

Bystander parents have challenges with detecting situations that will require parental attention. Bystander parents need a lot of sensory input themselves, and so cues that would indicate potential danger might go unnoticed. The Bystander parent might also miss their child's attempts to get attention, or to get their needs met.

Tips

○ **Note: These children are quickly overwhelmed by sensory input so these ideas show how to manage sensory input for them.**

○ Create a set menu for the week and post it in the kitchen so you can talk about it; this enables you to stay focused and the child to predict what sensory input will occur.

○ Warm cleansing wipes before using them during diapering, or to clean hands and face; room temperature sensations are easier for the child to manage.

○ Make toys and other play materials easily accessible so the child doesn't get overwhelmed just getting toys together.

○ Put things away so there are less busy areas for the child to look at.

○ Select natural fibers such as cotton for clothing to control the sensations to the skin.

○ Purchase firm-fitting undershirts/panties because they provide even pressure on skin which is calming to the child's system.

○ Find getaway places at large family gatherings so the child can learn to manage the amount of sensory input during chaotic situations.

○ Give family members earphones for their music/TV/radio so the child doesn't have to deal with competing sounds.

○ Run a fan in the room to create an even background noise; this decreases the effect of unpredictable noises.

○ Use repetitive movements for calming (e.g. rocking, bouncing slowly, swaying).

○ Select heavy blankets for the child's bedding; this provides calming input for getting to sleep.

○ Provide backdrops for them to make play areas smaller and less distracting

○ Play even-tempo background music or radio so the child has predictable auditory input

Cracking the Sensory Code in Specific Areas of Living

Now that you know how to apply the sensory code in the routines of everyday life, it is time to tackle special areas of life. Your sensory patterns can have a strong influence on these aspects of life because they introduce special circumstances you have to manage. You may discover that you have different reactions in one or another part of life because of what that activity demands from you. Understanding the sensory system within these life situations makes you even better able to manage your sensory needs successfully.

- o Chapter 7 deals with the special circumstances that food presents, including eating, dining out, and cooking, with all the associated smells, tastes, textures, and variety of eating places.

- o Chapter 8 addresses the special demands that clothing places on people. Fabrics, undergarments, and accessories can affect a person's reactions during the day and the right clothing for you can improve your life immensely.

- o Chapter 9 looks at living spaces, including what type of floor plan, furniture arrangements, and decorations will be most pleasant for people with different sensory patterns.

- o Chapter 10 deals with the special circumstances of work. People don't always have control over their workspaces, meeting patterns, and so on, so managing sensory needs in this situation can really help work productivity.

- o Chapter 11 considers the special situations of leisure. This is the most personal part of our lives, where we get to choose how to recharge our batteries, so designing and selecting activities that are respectful of sensory needs is critical to feeling rejuvenated.

7

Hungry? Let Your Senses Lead the Way!

The experience of making and eating food is a complex process that includes emotional, psychological, developmental, physical, and social features. On a biological level, food is fuel for human beings; we need it to survive and thrive. However, food also contributes to other aspects of our experiences as human beings. Food provides a way for people to gather and spend time together. When we meet for a meal, we have time to get to know each other better while dining. For those who like to cook, food provides a way to release tension, express creativity, and explore sensory experiences.

Opening story

The "favorite" home-cooked meal

The Wells family has many family stories they like to share. Because there are six people in the core family (parents and four children), their recollections of childhood events don't always match (well, if the truth be told, they *rarely* match). As adults, the storytelling has become legendary, with the family members' partners serving as a brand new audience for the banter.

The mother particularly enjoys stories about meal time and food. While they were raising their children, she made many home-cooked meals that would be sure to fill up her hungry crowd. A regular week night meal was chicken and dumplings. Mom is fascinated by different family members' description of this frequent meal.

Louise is the oldest. Chicken and dumplings was her favorite meal growing up. Here is how Louise describes this meal:

> I can still virtually experience the chicken and dumplings that my mother made for us; the creamy aroma of the chicken broth as the meat cooked with the celery and onions; the heat that emanated from the pot when Mother sifted out the chicken parts to make room for the long, thick, flat, wide, sticky home-made noodles. My hands were dry with the flour, and then became gluey as we dropped the noodles into the broth. I remember they had to cook for 14 minutes. During that time we could hear the gurgling as the air tried to escape from the broth, thickening with the flour from the noodles, the air oozed between the noodles to reach the surface and explode. When Mother served it to us, she poured the broth, noodles, and meat over cubes of potatoes; every version of beige (the one color thing bugged me a little). I am salivating just telling you this story; the hot broth coating my mouth and throat, the contrast of textures in the firm potatoes, the chewy noodles, and the softened meat from all that cooking. I can still feel the strings in the pieces of celery, even though they gave way in my mouth since they had been cooked so long.

Derek is one of the middle brothers, and he can hardly let Louise finish as she reverently recalls her experience:

> OK, so it cooked in a pot just like all our soups and stews. And technically Louise is correct about the description of the meal. But her *swooning* as she talks about it makes me want to gag. I would do *anything* to get out of touching the noodle batter; Mom thought I was "just a boy" who thought it wasn't cool to cook. I just didn't want all that icky stuff on my hands. When we got our bowls to eat, the noodles were slimy on the outside, and dense on the inside, so it was a nightmare to manage them in my mouth. I usually mashed it all up with my fork so I wouldn't have to contend with all those changes in my mouth. The chicken didn't mash too well, so I tried to work around the strands of meat.

Sam, the youngest son, is fascinated by all this discussion because he barely remembers any differences in their childhood meals:

Wow, you guys were way too focused on these mind-numbing details! I was just *hungry*. I remember that I got full, and that we had a lot of meals with all the food cooked together in the pot…that's all.

Which family member sounds more like you? Which family member reminds you of someone in your family? Although all of us have experiences such as this one, and we might even remember similar features of those experiences, we might not have the same reactions to those experiences.

Introduction

Think about your responses to food experiences. These responses will indicate your sensory patterns related to cooking, eating, and dining out. Think of the bread industry as it has tried to deal with the conflict between wholegrain and wheat breads compared with white bread. Children in particular prefer white bread because of its look (white), texture (soft, spongy), and taste (sweet). Wholegrain bread is brown, rough ("you can feel the seeds") and sharp (all the reasons some people love wholegrain bread!).

The lists below provide some examples of responses that suggest each sensory processing pattern in the food area. Identify your sensory pattern (and those of your family and friends!) when food is involved.

You are a Seeker in food situations if you:

o enjoy a wide range of foods

o experiment with recipes

o enjoy multiple course meals

o add unusual and varied spices to foods

o include others in cooking activities

o enjoy active, busy restaurants

o select busy times to eat at restaurants

o enjoy active dining experiences (e.g. preparing foods at the table)

o want large groups of family and friends dining together

o choose dining experiences that include entertainment

o create a "center of the party" atmosphere.

You are an Avoider in food situations if you:

- o have a set menu at home
- o are comfortable eating alone, and sometimes even prefer it
- o turn down more dining invitations than you accept
- o order the same food item every time you go to a specific restaurant
- o ask for sauces to be omitted from a menu item
- o lobby for off-peak dining times with your friends
- o have a list of foods you reject from your life.

You are a Bystander in food situations if you:

- o are satisfied with many dining options
- o are surprised to hear others' comments about foods because you hadn't thought of them
- o let others choose dining options
- o eat when others mention it is time to eat
- o only notice textures, tastes, or temperatures of food when others mention it
- o lose track of conversations during long meals
- o forget ingredients in recipes when cooking
- o forget dishes that you prepared and left in the fridge or on the stove
- o prefer others to do the planning and preparation.

You are a Sensor in food situations if you:

- o regularly make changes in menu items when ordering in a restaurant
- o send food back to get it "fixed"/prepared to suit your exacting needs
- o ask for special seating out of the way in restaurants
- o select specific recipes with only preferred ingredients
- o follow recipes precisely

○ choose quieter restaurants

○ prefer off-peak times to dine in restaurants.

From birth, we have a social and psychological relationship with food. We relate to the person who feeds us as infants and toddlers, since we cannot obtain food for ourselves. Food is social because of the interaction between the baby and the care provider; we begin to derive meaning from the experience of being fed, and becoming satisfied. As we grow, the experience of feeding someone, being fed, eating alone, and with others adds more layers to the meaning of food in our lives. Because initially we need help getting nourishment, food also takes on meaning related to feeling full, being hungry, getting needs met (or not), being taken care of, or being abandoned.

So when we talk about food, we have to look at the overall picture. The sensory processing aspects of food are very important, and we have to avoid the trap of thinking that sensory processing is the answer to every issue people have about eating. Considering sensory processing merely provides one more way to understand our reactions to food and eating is an essential part of everyday life.

We all have stories we can tell about ourselves, family members, friends, or even strangers in relation to some eating or dining out experience. Perhaps you grew up with a sibling who was a picky eater, or a parent who never wanted to eat out. Perhaps from your perspective, you have a friend or partner who over-spices (or under-spices) food.

Maybe more than any other daily life activity, food brings out our unique sensory tendencies. Understanding the sensory meaning of our choices can be extremely helpful as we decide where, with whom, and what we eat. When we observe people doing "weird" things related to food and eating, they are showing what their sensory needs and preferences are. When the people around you can understand why you are doing something, there is a greater chance that they will understand you better too.

General factors to consider in food experiences

There are four general factors to consider when thinking about the impact of sensory patterns on our eating experiences. Where you eat (settings), who you eat with (social context), what you eat (food choices), and how you prepare your own food (cooking) are all important aspects of food experiences.

Selecting locations for eating and dining out

You eat every day, probably in a variety of locations. Some locations are satisfying for you, others may be neutral, and still others may be unpleasant places for eating. Most of us get to select the location for eating and dining out some of the time, but not all of the time. When you understand what aspects of a setting are supportive to your style of sensory processing, you can guide group choices, design optimal choices for yourself, or make simple adaptations to improve the settings in which you find yourself eating and dining out.

> Think about the layout, lighting, background sounds, and fragrances when selecting a place for eating and dining out

When considering the sensory processing features of your dining locations, think about the layout of the space (see Chapter 9), lighting, background music, ambient noise, fragrances from the kitchen, and type of seating. For example, you are at a bustling bistro, with a strong garlic aroma and background string music. This setting will be inviting for those of you who are Seekers, yet may be overwhelming for an Avoider.

Social contexts for dining out and eating

Meal time is not just a time for obtaining nourishment. It is also a time for interacting with others. When we fail to acknowledge this important contextual feature of dining, we miss opportunities to make the most of meal time situations. We can have the physical context set up just right to meet our needs and still experience challenges because the truth is that people also generate sensory experiences for us as we interact with them, or even if they are in our surrounding environment. Talking, sitting, or standing close by, moving about a room, wearing cologne, and clothing choices of others can affect us during eating experiences.

> Talking, sitting, standing close, moving around the room, wearing cologne, and clothing choices can all affect dining experiences

Food selection

Foods provide an abundance of sensory experiences. Not only do they have taste, texture, and aromas in their natural state, we can adjust the sensory qualities of foods when we cook them. Then we have spices and sauces we can add to foods, condiments and toppings, and heat and cold to adjust the natural characteristics of foods. So food options can be both a great way to manage our sensory needs, and provide an assault to our systems when the foods contain characteristics that are hard for us to manage.

The box below contains actual descriptions people have made for the three foods; think about your own reactions to the following:

Descriptions of foods and *your* reactions

Food	Descriptions	Your reaction
Pear	grainy, like sugary sand	
	juicy, wet	
	sweet and soft	
Cooked mushrooms	soft, rubbery	
	warm and wet	
	bitter, earthy	
	squeaky on your teeth	
Italian bread	crunchy, chewy on the outside	
	soft and airy on the inside	
	uneven texture	
	bitter, yeasty	

You probably agree with many of the descriptions of these foods. The question relevant to sensory processing is "How do you *feel* about these characteristics?" Some people will find "grainy," "rubbery," and "yeasty" to be interesting, while others will be disgusted by them. Some people won't eat cooked mushrooms because of these characteristics, while others will make sure to add them *because* of these characteristics. Your sensory responses will affect your diet and food choices, and conversely, can give insights about your sensory preferences.

Cooking as part of the food experience

How people decide to prepare food reflects their sensory patterns. When people cook from scratch, many of the decisions are based on their sensory needs. For example, chopping raw vegetables and stirring thick sauces provide intense sensory input (the resistance as you chop and stir provides sensory input to the muscles and joints; the smells of the food as they are chopped and stirred; the sounds of the utensils; the visual changes in the foods as they change form). For some people, these activities are very satisfying (e.g. for Seekers), while for others, these actions are exhausting (e.g. for Avoiders). More complex food preparation is likely to be attractive to Seekers because of the variety of sensory experiences available in the cooking. Avoiders in cooking are more likely to have a few simple favorite recipes. Sensors in cooking will select recipes with their same favorite ingredients. Bystanders may forget to include an ingredient while cooking, or miss a step in the process.

> Food preparation is a sensory
> experience; some people enjoy these
> sensory experiences, while others find them exhausting

Let's consider how people with each type of sensory processing can make the most out of their eating and dining out experiences.

Seekers in eating and dining out situations

You know from earlier chapters that Seekers want a lot of interesting sensory experiences in their lives. There are no better daily activities than those related to food to enrich the Seeker's life. Let's consider John.

John loves going to the neighborhood Indian restaurant; it is a favorite of many people in the area. He can smell the spices as he walks down the sidewalk. The restaurant is decorated with many artifacts from India, and the tables have multicolor cloths with gold threads woven in. It is a small room, so everyone is close together while waiting for a table and when seated. He loves seeing everyone's food as it is delivered to neighboring tables, and sometimes asks other customers what they are having. He likes to order multiple dishes so he can have multiple flavors during the evening.

Seekers will enjoy loud, active, busy restaurants, especially town favorites that ensure that there will be lots of activity in the waiting area and lots to see, hear, and experience during the meal. Seekers might select dining experiences, such as dinner theatre, large buffets, or dinner dancing situations. If you are a Seeker, you will enjoy restaurants that cook at the table such as Japanese steakhouses. Seekers are also attracted to dining establishments that have large collections of objects adorning the walls and ceilings, creating a menagerie or flea market effect.

Seekers want intense sensory experiences during meals. Having a crowd gathered together for meals, encouraging people to banter at the table, interrupting each other, and being animated in their conversations would be a great experience for Seekers. The complexity of cocktails and appetizers in one room, and then moving into another room for the meal, is exciting because this situation provides a continuous flow of new sensory inputs. Seekers are also likely to create or select settings that have background music during eating, to increase the sensory intensity of the overall dining experience. When entertaining, people who seek sensation will seat people next to unfamiliar guests to increase the opportunities for interaction. People who seek sensation enjoy being the center of party environments, changing conversation topics, and raising provocative issues during the meal time. It is certainly true that these are social activities, but when looking at them from a sensory point of view, they also create opportunities for more unusual, intense sensory input.

At home, you might want the TV or stereo to be on, leave the food in the kitchen affording an opportunity to get up for seconds, and may select different places to sit and eat during a week (e.g. on the couch, sitting on the floor, at the table, at the counter). The additional complications of holding the plate, utensils, and drink make the eating experience more interesting. If you are a Seeker, you might also have multiple sets of dishes, place mats, and napkins, which is an easy way to create new experiences as you mix and match pieces together at different meals.

Seekers want interesting and noticeable foods. Therefore, ethnic foods are a common selection for Seekers. Seekers will also enjoy varied textures and flavors, and will want to experiment with unfamiliar spices when dining out and when cooking at home. If you are a Seeker, you will also enjoy having hot and cold items at the same meal, and may want to serve those foods in several different dishes to keep their features distinct throughout the meal. Tapas, multiple appetizers, and multiple-course food selection alternatives will be very inviting for you if you are a Seeker. You will also want spices and sauces at the table to alter your food as you eat.

Seekers can be adventurous cooks. Seekers will try new recipes frequently, and will be intrigued about finding new spices or ingredients. Seekers enjoy the food preparation process because it provides so many different sensory experiences, and they last so long! There are sounds from utensils and appliances, smells as food cooks, continuously changing visual images as food is mixed, layered, and transformed, and lots of movement around the room to get to cabinets, refrigerator, stove, and dishwashers. If you are brave enough to venture into the kitchen when a Seeker is hard at work, brace yourself for a wild ride! Seekers are also likely to make a big mess in the kitchen; they don't need to keep cleaning as they go because the clutter keeps the kitchen interesting.

Seekers who are not cooks might add spices or sauces to prepared foods. They might also serve prepared foods on decorative plates to make the meal more interesting visually.

Here are some suggestions for Seekers in food situations to make their experiences more satisfying.

Seekers can make food situations more satisfying if they:

o choose loud, active, busy restaurants during heavy-use times so the noise and activity can keep their interest

o select restaurants that prepare foods at the table to keep things changing during the meal

o suggest buffet dining so they can move around during the meal

o include larger groups of people in their dining parties so they can shift from one conversation to another during the meal

o dine in combination with entertainment so they can shift their attention from the food to the entertainment and back again

o try different ethnic foods, and cook with unusual spices to keep their flavor and taste interests peaked

o combine foods with different textures, or cold and hot foods at the same meal to stimulate changes during the meal

o keep spices such as pepper sauce at the table so they can adjust the spiciness experience throughout the meal.

Bystanders in eating and dining situations

Bystanders will do better in a more changeable environment for meals. When things are changing around them, Bystanders can pay attention better during the meal. However, not all meals require a high degree of attention; in these cases, any environment will be acceptable to Bystanders.

If you are a Bystander for eating, then meals with several courses are great; the activity of clearing the place and refilling it with the next course creates activity and interest. There are sounds, aromas, sights associated with serving each course, and these additional sensory experiences create the extra input you need to stay completely aware of the meal and your meal partners.

Another good option is the self-serve venue. Getting up frequently takes advantage of movement and muscle activity to keep you focused on the meal and on the people you are dining with. If you have a choice, select seating in the traffic pattern of the entrance, kitchen, or bathrooms to increase the activity around you during the meal as well. Noticing people going by is a natural way to keep you alert.

When dining at home, change where you eat your meals during the week and keep the food in the kitchen, so if you want more, you have to get up to get it. Consider having plates, bowls, and place mat sets in different patterns, so you have different place settings on different days. At work, get up and move to a new location for lunch or snacks, even if it is down the hall or in the lobby. The movement will activate you with more sensory input (e.g. movement, visual changes, sounds), and a busier location will provide additional input while eating. Go with colleagues to the cafeteria or other busy locations for your meal times.

Bystanders will also need contrast and variety in their foods because this will keep you more alert during the meal. Bystanders might not remember to select these items, and may need to be reminded, either by friends and family, or by reminding yourself (e.g. a note card on the cabinet door).

CHANGE IT UP! Colors, flavors, temperatures, textures, smells... YOU CAN HAVE IT ALL!

Bystanders need to select foods that require different utensils. For example, include meat or vegetables that need to be cut up, and serve applesauce or cottage cheese that needs to be scooped. Put serving bowls on the table so you have to serve yourself during the meal. Multiple colors, textures, temperatures, and flavors of food will all help maintain your attention while eating. Place condiments on the table, such as peppers, mustards, and vinegars, to provide both flavors and the opportunity to interact with foods while eating.

Bystanders are easy-going cooks; they don't feel pressure to be precise with their measurements, procedures, or the timing. If something turns out funny, Bystanders will shrug or laugh it off rather than get stressed out about it. Bystanders might miss ingredients, or add something twice because they didn't recall adding it the first time. This is what happened to Rachel.

Rachel was just learning how to cook, and was enjoying herself. She found a recipe for bran muffins that were great for her to make before she left for the school bus every day because she could make a big batch of the batter and keep it in the refrigerator all week. Then each morning she just had to bake the muffins she wanted for that morning; she loved them being fresh each day. On Wednesday morning of the first week, Rachel's brother asked if he could have a couple of muffins with her. Rachel was delighted, and prepared muffins from the batter for both of them. When they came out of the oven piping hot, she proudly served them with jam. Thomas took one bite and gagged. "This is like biting into the salt shaker," he said. Rachel didn't know what he was talking about since she had been eating muffins for two days already. Mom came into the kitchen to find out what was going on, and Thomas made her taste the muffins. Mom agreed that the muffins were very salty. Rachel hadn't noticed the flavor, and Mom figured she had put the salt ingredient in more than once to get the batter that salty.

Rachel is a Bystander. She added the salt more than once, and didn't taste the intensely salty flavor when she ate the muffins. Her ability to detect flavor intensity was very low compared with other family members.

Bystanders need the intensity of sensory experiences during meal times; they are not as likely to generate these opportunities for themselves (Rachel is the exception with the extra salt!). In order to stay connected to the social aspect of the dining experience, Bystanders need to be either in naturally busy environments, or need cues that will keep them active throughout. At a meal, seating placement in the middle of the table provides more opportunities for passing food, turning left and right to interact with others, and being physically close to others.

At a party, a Bystander will do better socially by selecting a location near high activity, such as near the food table or near the door, because these locations are ever-changing and therefore will provide an intense sensory background. With an intense sensory background, Bystanders can remain attentive and engaged with others at the party. It is also helpful for Bystanders to sit or stand near a person who is more likely to direct the conversation because enthusiastic talkers provide multisensory cues and invite continuous responses. Bystanders are good at engaging in focused discussion during busy experiences; Bystanders are not distracted by the things going on around them. This skill makes them good conversation partners.

The list below provides a summary of suggestions for making eating and dining out the best it can be for Bystanders.

Bystanders can make food situations more satisfying if they:

- o make sure there is enough lighting and background noise to support attention and awareness in the dining experience

- o choose restaurants that serve multiple courses so that the continuous changes at the table can keep attention during the meal

- o select buffets and self-serve locations so there are many opportunities to get up and move around

- o dine with people who will direct the conversation so they can stay attentive to what is happening at the table

- o stand at the door or near the food table at parties so there are many interruptions to keep their attention on what is going on around them

- o place contrasting colors of food on plate to increase its visual interest

- o use family-style dining at home, so everyone is passing dishes and serving themselves throughout the meal

- o provide vinegars, pepper sauces, and other herbs at the dinner table to increase the variety of food experiences at the table

- o create contrasting flavors (e.g. sweet and sour), temperatures, and textures for the table.

Sensors in eating and dining situations

Sensors are highly likely to notice characteristics of eating and dining environments. Sensors detect aromas, notice volume of ambient noise, and take note of particular characteristics of chairs or seating arrangements. It will be useful for you to identify favorite restaurants in your community; you can select them based on your personal preferences for flavors and aromas, but there are also other considerations that may make your outings more enjoyable. For example, off-peak hours provide a calmer sensory environment and therefore won't overwhelm you quite so easily. Restaurants that are more dimly lit, or that have a more sedate or romantic atmosphere, may be more desirable. Also, ask to be seated at the edge of the rooms, in a contained space, and out of traffic patterns; these choices reduce the possibility of being bombarded with random sensory input that occurs in the normal course of eating out.

Andrew is studying to be a wine sommelier, and has received accolades for his skill at noticing the characteristics of wines. He is so happy to have found this path for his career because as a child there were battles with his mother regarding his constant comments about foods. Andrew would notice that his mother forgot the oregano, or cooked the sauce to a different texture from the last time. Learning about the characteristics of wines channeled this detailed awareness into a very satisfying kind of work. As a Sensor for taste, smell, and texture, Andrew has the potential to detect more details about the wines, and therefore to be a more gifted sommelier.

There may be days when you feel too "filled up" with sensory input to manage dining in a restaurant. On these days, Sensors may do better with carry-out foods so you can choose a more manageable location. Although home may be an option, you might also select a quiet area of a building or park.

Wendy and Saira are dear friends. They met through their work, but have become personal friends as well. They have a "date" to catch up over dinner once a month. They always go to one of Saira's favorite local restaurants because Saira knows the menus have selections she likes, and the menus are broad enough to give Wendy some variety. These restaurants are also small, so there is a predictable amount of activity, especially since they tend to go to dinner earlier than other people.

Wendy loves catching up with Saira's life, but she also loves dining with her because she knows she will get extra vegetables every time they eat out. Saira always orders one of two meal options (usually the steak), and will only eat the meat and the mashed potatoes. No matter how the vegetables are prepared, Saira will not venture into the vegetable world. She says she doesn't like green things, and then goes on to describe the way they feel in her mouth. "They seem cooked, and then sometimes there is this dense center that surprises you; you can't tell how they will break up in your mouth." Wendy laughs because she *totally* agrees with Saira's descriptions; it is just that Wendy *loves* all those things about vegetables!

Sensors identify a set of favorite foods and select them regularly. These favorite foods will share some important characteristics, such as similar textures, tastes, smells, and flavors, because a person who is sensitive will reject many other options for food. Sensors will notice even small changes in a recipe, such as an increase in a spice, pasta being cooked less (or more), or fruit being just a little more ripe than desired. Sensors also notice the temperature at which food is served, and are likely to prefer foods closer to room temperature.

Sensors prefer to plan eating and dining out experiences carefully. Since Sensors can be overwhelmed by sensory input, crowded places with lots of people can sometimes provide too much input, making an otherwise pleasant eating experience more challenging. Sensors select social dining situations with small groups of people, frequently with familiar friends and family. When people are familiar, they are more predictable from a sensory point of view (e.g. you know what their cologne smells like, you know the movements of their gestures, you know the sounds of their laughter, thereby reducing the chances of being bombarded by unfamiliar or unpredictable input). When the social environment is more predictable, then dining can take center stage of the person's attention and focus. Sensors will enjoy more strategic locations, like the end of the table, or near the edges of the room at a cocktail party, so they can participate while reducing the random input of central locations.

This doesn't mean that people with sensitivity will never be in crowded social dining situations. However, when life calls for participating in a busier social situation, Sensors will need to prepare for the experience, and will likely need quiet time afterward to regroup to a calm state. Unlike Seekers, who are energized by complex social situations, Sensors may be depleted and need rest afterwards.

When cooking, Sensors maintain their precise focus on details in an effort to make sure all their food and eating requirements are met. Sensors have favorite recipes, spices, presentation styles; it is easy to tell their preferences because they reoccur in all their foods and meals. Sensors who are cooks can be very bossy in the kitchen, as you can see in Wolfgang's story.

Wolfgang is cherished by his friends and family and yet he can be so exasperating! He is very passionate in the kitchen, but his friends and family have learned to make themselves scarce while he is cooking. He is very precise about the preparation, including wanting uniform sizes in the onion and garlic pieces, and measuring spices very carefully. No one meets

Wolfgang's standards, and so there are tense moments in the kitchen when friends and family try to help. Everyone reaps the rewards of his love of cooking as long as they haven't been around him while he is cooking.

Wolfgang can be an insufferable dining partner as well. When he has not been the cook, he doesn't know exactly how the food was prepared, so he analyzes every detail of the foods, including the textures, temperatures, flavors, color, and even presentation. He has an uncanny ability to detect the spices in sauces, and wants others at the table to taste the food and analyze the spices with him. His friends love the flavor of the food, and urge him just to enjoy the experience, but he persists with his analysis games.

In restaurants, Wolfgang is infamous for sending plates back to have the foods warmed "properly" or to adjust the spice in a dish. He can detect the slightest amount of unevenness in creamy mashed potatoes, and will insist that others taste the foods to detect the same things he detects. His friends have learned which restaurants provide the most consistent food preparation for Wolfgang, and so tend to select the same neighborhood spots so they can have more of Wolfgang's quick wit and less of his intense "food detective" persona during an evening meal.

Wolfgang is a Sensor in eating and dining experiences. He has a highly developed ability to detect the details of sensory experiences in foods. His need for precision suggests that he notices even very small changes in sensory input; other people would not notice the differences in saltiness or creaminess until a bigger difference occurred. Sensors can become experts because of their detection abilities; Wolfgang is seen as a master of food by his friends and family.

The following list provides a summary of some suggestions for Sensors in food situations.

Sensors can make food situations more satisfying if they:

o dine during off-peak hours, at favorite restaurants so they know the routine and the menu

o ask for quiet, dark, and intimate restaurant locations so that the room does not overwhelm them

o request seating at the edge of the room, out of the traffic paths so they won't get bumped or bothered during the meal

o choose a small group of friends/family to dine with so they can track the conversation and won't be distracted o stand or sit at the edges of parties so they can visit with people without being overwhelmed

o identify their optimal flavors, temperatures (e.g. room temperature), and textures for foods so they can easily identify menu items and recipes that will be pleasing for them

o stick with favored spices and food preparation strategies so they will not be overwhelmed by their meal.

Avoiders in eating and dining situations

Avoiders select quiet, controlled environments for eating and dining out. They are most comfortable staying home where the sensory environment is predictable (light, sound, feel of chairs). Avoiders can prepare foods "just the right way" at home. Avoiders also order favorites for carry-out or home delivery. They can create a space for eating and dining that has comfortable seating, use plain pattern dishes and simple place mats or tablecloths. When the regular activity of eating is comfortable, you will have the resources to tackle other things in your day.

This does not mean that Avoiders will never go out to eat. Although Avoiders prefer the comforts of home (because this is a predictable sensory setting), preparing ahead for a restaurant experience makes it more manageable. Select local, familiar restaurants that have predictable patterns of service, and that have self-contained seating areas for small numbers of guests. Consider driving separately from your friends and family so you can leave when you feel overwhelmed without making everyone else join you. However, dining out doesn't always look like you think it might; Avoiders need to experiment with the exact characteristics of their low sensory thresholds. Consider Marion's story.

Marion and her husband make a plan to go out to eat about once a month. They have spent a lot of time negotiating about where they would eat so they both have an enjoyable time. At first, Marion pushed for going early so they would miss the crowds because she tends to get overwhelmed with crowded and noisy places. However, this didn't turn out as she had imagined. She says:

> When we went to these quiet restaurants in their "off" hours, we would be greeted by eager staff wanting to serve us. The staff really bugged me by coming over to the table so often; they would talk to us and

bump into me as they worked the table. Other staff would be standing around waiting for more people to show up, chatting with each other. The worst thing, though, was my dear husband Cliff. He is a noisy eater; he has a jaw that pops, and he makes other noises related to his sheer enjoyment of the food. In these quiet places I could hear every sound he made! Even though the place was romantic, this did not put me into a romantic mood at all.

Marion and Cliff finally found the perfect solution. Marion discovered that she could handle more background noise of a busier restaurant if they either had reservations (so they could be quiet at home beforehand) or if the restaurant had a separate and quiet waiting area while waiting to be seated. The higher noise level inside the restaurant drowned out Cliff's eating sounds, and the staff were busier so they did not hover over their table. She learned that the general background noise was more even, and so didn't bother her as much.

So, Marion is an Avoider in public situations like restaurants. But she discovered that not every single aspect of the sounds and touch in these places was overwhelming for her. She learned that specific, individual, and focused sounds were harder to manage than more general background noises. She learned that by getting some "quiet" time before the meal, she could manage more background noise for a period of time. Since she was motivated to spend time with her husband, these solutions made everything pleasant for both of them.

While out in the community or at work, it is sometimes harder to manage eating and dining out environments. When running errands, you may prefer drive-through food or carry-out items, or you may prefer to bring food along in your bag, so you don't have to contend with the demands of public dining while you are trying to get other things accomplished. At work, find a quiet place you can occupy for a few minutes to enjoy your meal or snack. This way, the challenges of more random eating environments (e.g. the cafeteria) will not deplete you for the rest of the work day.

People with sensation-avoiding patterns are more likely to have a routine menu for meals. You will like foods prepared in one way, and without additional sauces and spices. If you are an Avoider, you may also have some rituals related to your eating. For example, you may eat one thing at a time on your plate until it is gone, and then go to the next item rather than mixing the foods during the meal. You may prefer to have your food separated, i.e. not touching each other because the flavors or textures mixing is unpleasant for you. These rituals reduce stress during the meal.

Identify your favorite foods and preparation strategies, and stick with them; this will enable you to participate in social and other aspects of dining without getting too overwhelmed. In your family, have spices and sauces served at the table so others can add them and you can eat the food without extra spicing. Identify what the important characteristics of food are for you, and explain them to your family so they can meet your needs.

Matt and his wife Sonya have been involved in a battle of wills for quite a while in the kitchen. Sonya enjoys cooking, and has certain "musts" in the kitchen. Sonya thinks that a dish is not worth cooking if she hasn't sautéed onions and garlic to begin. "It just doesn't have any flavor without this base," she says.

At first, Matt was so in love with Sonya, he didn't say anything, and choked the food down. He even tells the story of their first date. He went over to Sonya's house for the first time, and she had made appetizers for them: *braised onion tarts!* Matt says the onions were snarled around each other and piled high on each tart like a nest of worms. And yet when he looked at Sonya's glowing and proud face, he couldn't do anything but eat one…and then another. He says that he never worked so hard not to gag.

When Matt first discussed the "I don't like onions" idea (he wanted to say I *detest onions*), Sonya was shocked. She said that onions were in every dish she made (as if Matt didn't already know). She reluctantly made a few dishes without any onions in them, and they both agreed that the flavor wasn't right. So with further discussion, Matt was able to figure out that it was the texture of cooked onions, not the flavor that bothered him. They went through some of their typical family dishes, and talked about them; sometimes Sonya would have big chunks of onion and other times the onions were smaller. Matt said that he could see and work around the big chunks; the flavor was still in the food from the onions, but he didn't have to contend with the texture of the onion in his mouth.

So now Sonya either pulverizes the onions so they are undetectable as a separate texture (more like onion paste), or she puts big chunks into her dishes so Matt can find them. They both feel satisfied and can even now laugh about their first date being such a challenging way to start their relationship!

You can also analyze the Sensory characteristics of the foods you are comfortable with (e.g. creamy), and identify other foods or preparation strategies that will broaden your selection while retaining those same important characteristics. For example, if you like creamy textures, you may dislike raw vegetables because of their crunchiness; you can find ways to prepare the vegetables to create a creaminess you like and expand your food choices. Balancing between what is tolerable for you and obtaining adequate nutrition is possible when you understand the Sensory characteristics of the foods you prefer.

Avoiders prefer dining alone or with one or two other people because this is a strategy for managing sensory input in the environment. At home, parents who are Avoiders in the food area might choose to dine after the children have been fed so their meal can be more quiet and structured. When attending parties, Avoiders do better if they stop by early and leave when it gets crowded, or attend later when the crowd has thinned. They may also need to eat before or after gatherings so they can focus on interacting with others and not have to worry about getting to the crowded food area. Avoiders are more likely to entertain in their homes, either cooking themselves or getting take-out food, so they have a predictable backdrop for their social interactions that revolve around dining (see Tom and Miranda's story in Chapter 5).

The following list provides a summary of some suggestions for Avoiders in the food and eating area.

Avoiders can make food situations more satisfying if they:

o eat at home most of the time so they can control the amount of input they have to manage at one time

o order carry-out or get home delivery rather than eating in the restaurant so they don't have to deal with all the noise and activity in the restaurant

o identify neighborhood restaurants with preferred menu items so they don't have to worry about what to order and can focus on the friend they are dining with

o dine with one other person or a small intimate group of people so they can focus on them without competing sounds and interruptions

o eat with partner after the children have eaten so they can concentrate on the children and then on their partner, which reduces interruptions

- o stop by very early and leave parties when they get crowded so they can honor their friends without becoming overwhelmed

- o create a routine menu for the week so they know what they will be experiencing along the way

- o use simple cooking methods such as steaming, roasting, and broiling so that foods have their own flavor without competing flavors from spices or sauces.

Dining is a family affair

Eating at home every day is what we experience the most. Negotiating everyone's sensory needs during dinner makes for an interesting evening. Let's look at one family and how they manage this situation.

Miriam rushes in the door of her home with her daughter Tracy in tow. She has about an hour to get dinner on the table for her family. She calls out to her teenager Felicity, who arrived home a little earlier, but has trouble getting Felicity's attention because her music is loud; she is on her cell phone, and Miriam hears the clicking of the computer keyboard. She tosses her bags onto the bench, and gets to work in the kitchen. She is grateful that Tracy has TV shows to watch so she doesn't have to entertain her six-year-old while she is trying to cook.

Arthur gets home about an hour later, just in time for dinner with his wife and daughters. Arthur and Miriam have had a vision of the perfect family meal time, but as they live the experience of eating dinner together, things work out quite differently. They have to pry Tracy away from the TV, and she is so entranced that she is like a zombie when she comes to the table. When she gets to the table, she lies on the table, drapes herself on her chair, and seems barely conscious. She not only doesn't talk to other family members, she also messes around with her food, and her parents get frustrated that she doesn't eat a balanced meal.

Felicity is happy to have a chance to eat. However, her parents have had to restrict her from using her cell phone at the table. They have also had to negotiate about what music plays in the background during the meal. They agreed to "music without words" to reduce the number of times that Felicity would burst out singing during dinner.

Miriam and Arthur try to have discussions about the day; Tracy doesn't even act like she knows her parents have asked her something. Felicity is less predictable. Some days, she answers "Nothing," "I don't know," and other cryptic responses when her parents ask her questions. Other days, she doesn't wait for an invitation to talk, and seems to be on an overly active autopilot, as stories about her friends and her day spill all over the table.

Miriam and Arthur have a much easier job meeting Felicity's needs than Tracy's. They let her have her time before dinner, talking on the phone, using the computer, and listening to music, so she is "loaded up" with sensory input by the time she comes to the table. She loves food, and Miriam is a creative cook, so Felicity has lots of smells, textures, and tastes to satisfy herself during the meal. Mom and dad talk continuously, and since they serve the meal family-style, Felicity has repeated opportunities to pass food to others. The family plays music in the background as well. All of these things keep Felicity's sensory systems activated throughout the meal.

Interestingly, many of the things Miriam and Arthur are doing have the potential to be helpful to Tracy too. Since she is a Bystander, Tracy needs extra sensory input just like Felicity as a Seeker. The problem is that Tracy has been watching TV, and has been very inactive for the hour before dinner. They decide to change some things to get Tracy back in the dinner game.

When mom gets home, instead of letting Tracy go to the TV, she gets her involved in the kitchen. She tells Tracy that her first job is to figure out what they are having for dinner. Tracy has to open the refrigerator, lift pot lids, and search on the counters for clues. She gets to smell the aromas, feel the steam or cold air on her face and hands, and mom encourages her to stir things and do "taste tests." Then mom and Tracy decide how to set the table, getting plates and place mats that contrast to the foods for the evening, and then Tracy gets the table ready. Mom gets out the food coloring and lets Tracy change the color of her milk with the appropriate droplets. At the table, they have guessing games about what spices are in the foods. With all the preparation activities, Tracy is activated as she comes to the dinner table, and with focused discussion about the food and meal, she is much more involved with her family during dinner.

When parents understand the sensory needs of their children, they can adjust everyday life activities to make them more satisfying for everyone.

8

Sensational Wardrobes

Clothing industry gurus have known for a long time that perfect clothing makes a difference in people's lives. It's just that people don't agree about what "perfect clothing" is. These individual differences can be understood by examining sensory patterns. Some people love loose clothing, while others adore a firm, tight fit — one that hugs and stays in place. Others want wool blends to keep warm, and others think wool is just too scratchy. What this translates into for designers and retailers is not only offering a range of sizes, designs, and colors, but also different fits, fabric, and textures to meet everyone's needs. The sensory patterns provide a basis for understanding different wardrobe preferences and choices.

Opening story

Clothing makes all the difference!

Hannah is *very* particular about her clothing:

> I do not like to wear heavy clothes or jewelry; I feel too weighted down. I won't wear cotton sweaters because they are too heavy and prefer light weight polar fleece instead. When I feel weighted down, I can't concentrate on other things I need to get done.

Hannah is a Sensor with her wardrobe, especially related to touch, and this affects what she is comfortable wearing. It doesn't take very much input for Sensors to feel overwhelmed. Since Hannah's work demands that she accomplishes lots of tasks during the day, it's important she minimizes basic sensory input, such as the sensations from her clothing, which then makes it possible for her to concentrate on her work and other activities. By selecting lightweight clothing and very little jewelry, she can concentrate on her daily tasks without discomfort or distraction.

But Chelsea is quite different. As a Seeker, she is particularly partial to firm touch on her skin. Unlike Hannah, Chelsea needs sensory input to keep herself organized and functioning at an optimal level. Just listen to her describe such needs:

> I love to be able to feel my clothing. I love to layer my clothes and wear a lot of accessories so that I can feel my skin all day long. It gives me the feeling of being grounded, and lets me know where my body ends and the world begins. I had to give an important talk before a large audience a couple of years ago, and I chose to wear a heavily beaded top under my suit because it made me feel anchored and calmer during the talk. Because I could feel the edge of my body very clearly, I could free my mind to concentrate on delivering my talk successfully.

As a Seeker, Chelsea selects clothing options that provide additional input because she needs more input to keep herself organized. By creating a constant background of input (i.e. wearing heavy, firm clothing), Chelsea doesn't have to create more input during activities. So instead of seeking more input through fiddling or jiggling in her chair, or pacing while talking to her colleagues to get the additional input she needs, she can focus on her work. She wears clothes that naturally give her input so she can proceed through her day, focused and confident.

So, Chelsea needs to have more sensory input to her skin so she can concentrate, while Hannah needs less sensory input to concentrate. Chelsea and Hannah seem to understand their own needs so they can structure their respective wardrobes to support their daily tasks. A "sensational wardrobe" is different for each of them.

Introduction

When we think about wardrobes, we think about style and function. Style includes the design of clothing items, the color, texture, and fabrics, the way people put their clothing together, and how people choose to accessorize. Function includes comfort, usefulness in particular situations, the image people want or need to portray, and the amount of protection the clothing provides. Style and function complement each other, and with a little planning, everyone can have a stylish and functional wardrobe.

Style is about sensation, not trends

Learning about sensory patterns introduces an additional factor to consider when creating a wardrobe that is just right for each person. Although the phrase "sensational dressing" triggers images of a person with high style, when meeting your sensory needs is a factor, "sensational dressing" means creating a wardrobe that provides satisfaction and comfort all day long. Clothing contacts the skin, regulates body temperature, can make noises, has texture, weight, brightness, contrast, movement, and can even have an aroma. So when we delve into our wardrobes, we probe into an intense sensory world that can either make our day incredible or treacherous.

> Sensational dressing means creating a wardrobe that provides satisfaction and comfort all day long

The definition of a "sensational wardrobe" is different for people with each pattern of sensory processing. If you wear something that looks "trendy" and you are pulling at your clothing all day, this won't look very trendy or stylish. People need to feel good in their clothing as part of being stylish; how people act in clothing can make a difference in both appearance and the impression others have as well. Creating options that meet your sensory needs can make your "trendy" choices more successful.

There are three aspects of clothing that are affected the most by sensory characteristics. Clothing is made of materials that have sensory qualities; accessories provide weight, sound, and visual characteristics, and undergarments are powerful because they touch the skin. Let's examine the sensory aspects of clothing with these three areas in mind.

Color, texture, and fabrics offer sensory options

The marketplace offers consumers a wide array of colors and textures in clothing, and it is more acceptable than ever for people to demonstrate their individuality when dressing for business, dining out, running errands, exercising, and attending other community events. People who are sensitive to fibers in wool can choose cotton or blended fabrics. Seekers can select many textures and colors for one outfit, while Avoiders can create a perfectly crafted monochromatic outfit. Bystanders can profit from lines of clothing that are dyed to match and coordinate with each other because this takes the guesswork out of getting an outfit put together.

Think about five favorite items in your wardrobe. What do these items have in common? Are they the same texture, color, or cut? Do they match each other or represent variety? This simple activity can help identify what factors might matter the most in your wardrobe. Some people are focused on the colors, wanting the visual experience to be a certain way. Other people will feel the fabrics to see how their skin might react. Each of these preferences reflects a personal sensory pattern that can guide wardrobe planning.

Accessories can be friends or foes to your senses

As illustrated in the opening story, accessories can be helpful or challenging as well. Chelsea needed more accessories to load up her sensory systems, while Hannah needed less to keep from overwhelming her senses. Not everyone is as aware of their sensory needs as Chelsea and Hannah. Many of us will be uncomfortable without realizing what is contributing to the "icky" feeling.

The opening story was about women's accessories. Men have to contend with accessories too. Fit of shoes and socks, belts, ties, and even cufflinks can contribute to a good or bad feeling all day. The same basic principles apply; if you need more sensory input from your clothing (i.e. as Seekers and Bystanders do), firm, heavy accessories will be more satisfying. Select a heavier watchband, use cufflinks and add a sweater under suits. If you need less sensory input from your clothing (i.e. as Sensors and Avoiders do), use few accessories, or none at all. For example, use a light digital pocket watch, your cell phone, or clocks on community buildings to find the time so you don't have to contend with a watch band.

Undergarments make or break your day

Undergarments are the foundation of your wardrobe. When undergarments fit poorly, it is hard to concentrate on anything else. Just like other aspects of the wardrobe, what constitutes the perfect undergarments is different for everyone. Yet each of us knows what the perfect arrangement is, and usually knows pretty quickly when we don't have the perfect undergarment arrangement.

Close contact with the skin increases the sensory aspect of undergarments. As we discussed in Chapter 2, there are two categories of touch to the skin. The first one involves firm, even pressure on the skin. Touch-pressure provides good information about the body surface, and makes a map of your shape for your brain (your brain really wants to keep track of your body parts throughout the day!). The second category includes light touch (the ticklish kind of touch), pain, and temperature. This kind of touch provides good information about what needs attention, and what might be a signal for danger (e.g. it's *hot*, or it *hurts*) so you can act quickly to be safe.

So, people don't need to be alerted all day about undergarments! We want to put them on and forget about them, so we can concentrate on other things. You probably have had one of these *alerting* days with your undergarments; it can be very distracting. The clothing industry has begun removing tags and thin elastic bands in undergarments; they are opting to get rid of a noticeable input (that scratchy tag or piercing elastic that signals the alerting part of the system), and give you more opportunities to have organizing input to your skin.

The cool thing is that organizing input to your skin is helpful to everyone. Select undergarments that give *just the right amount of even pressure* to your skin. Bands or elastic that press more than the fabric around the band can make an uncomfortable place. Sometimes wider bands even out the pressure, and can be comfortable for people. When you find the ones that work for your sensory needs, you will be much happier.

The following lists can give you a general idea of which sensory patterns affect your wardrobe the most.

You are a Seeker in your wardrobe if you:

o have an eclectic, idiosyncratic style

o select bright colors and high contrasts in outfits

o prefer patterns in fabrics

- vary the textures of clothing

- enjoy a wide range of accessories.

You are an Avoider in your wardrobe if you:

- have a limited set of acceptable clothing items

- select firm-fitting clothing that doesn't move around on the body

- won't use accessories

- have undergarments in your drawer that you will not wear

- throw away wardrobe items after one wearing.

You are a Sensor in your wardrobe if you:

- are very picky about clothing choices because many items aren't exactly right

- feel or smell clothes on the rack to find acceptable fabrics

- get clothing items tailored to fit perfectly

- have a color palate that pervades your wardrobe

- wear solid colors

- wear light, sparse accessories.

You are a Bystander in your wardrobe if you:

- have an easy-going style

- spend very little time worrying about your wardrobe

- sometimes have two different socks on

- find yourself without accessories sometimes

- find your shirt buttoned unevenly occasionally.

Sensational wardrobes for seekers

Since Seekers always want more, the wardrobe is a great place to get more sensory information. Clothing and accessories have qualities that can provide a whole range of extra sensory input. Depending on what type of sensory input the Seeker wants, Seekers can select clothing and accessories that will meet those needs.

Sarah Jane is a middle school student who is running for class representative to the student council. She is very excited about this opportunity because it is her first time to try for a leadership spot with her classmates. When she gets home from school, Sarah Jane's mother wants to know how things went. Sarah Jane tells her mother everything that happened for the voting:

> So, Mom, there were five people running from our class alone. I am really glad that we practiced my speech last night, because some of the other kids didn't, and you could totally tell. After that, we sat down, and had to put our heads on the desk for voting, so we couldn't tell who was voting for which kid. That part was so lame, because even with my head down, I could tell who was voting for me because you can hear their clothing rubbing on itself when they raised their hands! Since I knew what people were wearing, it wasn't a secret at all! Why didn't Ms. Smythe think of that?

Seekers like Sarah Jane sometimes don't realize that others don't pay attention to sensory input the way they do. It doesn't occur to her that no one else knows what clothing sounds like, nor have very many others noticed what people are wearing. Probably Sarah Jane has picked out clothing preferences based on how the fabrics sound when she moves (won't her mother be interested in knowing this for future purchases?). Her need to seek more input has resulted in Sarah Jane having a lot more detailed information about clothing and fabric than anyone could have imagined!

Seekers for touch can select draped, textured fabrics, or tight fits, or even heavy jewelry, scarves, and hosiery. If a person seeks sound, then swishy fabrics, jewelry that clacks together, shoes with noisy soles or corduroy will do the trick. It is always important to remember that Seekers will have certain sensory inputs that are their favorites, and they will select wardrobe options to meet specific needs.

The Seeker's style is noticeable to everyone

The Seeker's style is likely to be noticeable to everyone. Seekers need more sensory input, so this will show up in their wardrobe. Seekers choose unusual wardrobe pieces and they may put items together in unusual ways. The process of mixing and matching satisfies the Seeker's need to add sensory input to dressing routines. Seekers put wardrobe items together in unique ways, and will not settle on one way. Imagine the stimulation for Seekers first thing in the morning, trying out different wardrobe pieces and accessories to find just the right look for that day. Seekers are more likely to become unsatisfied and bored with their wardrobe than others. Due to this, it is probably a good idea for Seekers to add cost-affordable accessories and trendy items to the wardrobe to satisfy the need for additional sensory input without breaking the bank.

Seekers will select wardrobe items with particular colors, textures, and fabrics to meet their particular needs. Seekers who want more touch will stroke their clothing throughout the day, so they will want nubby, slick, or rough textures in their clothing so they will have a zing of sensory input every time they touch their clothes. Seekers who want more visual input will select bright and high-contrast wardrobe items. Seekers who need more auditory input will select clothing and accessories that make noise. For example, corduroy makes a sound when you walk; varied textures rub against each other and make interesting sounds; clothing with sequins and beads makes a noise when the pieces bump together; heavy jewelry makes noises when the earrings, bracelets, and necklaces move. Shoes with wooden or thin leather heels, metal taps, tassels, thick ties, and no back strap make a myriad of sounds as you walk. Seekers who need pressure input to their muscles and joints will select heavy, layered clothing, carry heavy briefcases or purses, wear heavy-soled shoes (e.g. wingtips) and select heavy accessories like cufflinks, necklaces, and bracelets.

Undergarments are critical to comfort and satisfaction with your wardrobe. For Seekers, this means that undergarments need to be both comfortable and provide extra sensory input throughout the day. For example, a fitted camisole or a snug undershirt provides continuous sensory input, and when the person moves, these undergarments stay pressed against the skin, providing more input. Heavier fabrics are sometimes more satisfying for Seekers as well. Seekers notice and select undergarments by the type of fabric, for example, silk provides feedback because of its smooth feeling.

General tips for a sensational Seeker wardrobe

Clothing:

- Interesting and unusual combinations

    ◦ Layered.

Fabrics:

    ◦ high feedback fabrics (e.g. textured, visually interesting, noisy like corduroy)

    ◦ colorful and highly contrasting parts.

Accessories:

    ◦ bold, large, and heavy

    ◦ variable materials, including metal, wood, feathers

    ◦ multiple items at a time.

Undergarments:

    ◦ firm-fitting with support

    ◦ smooth textures.

Tips for creating a sensational Seeker wardrobe

    ◦ Select fabrics that have textures you can feel (velvet, cashmere, fur).

    ◦ Select fabrics that make a noise when you move (corduroy).

    ◦ Select accessories that are heavy, noisy, textured (feathers, beads that bump into each other, oversized belts and buckles, cufflinks).

    ◦ Include a wide range of shoe options to keep interest visually and from the touch of the shoes on the feet.

    ◦ Select undergarments that touch the skin in pleasant ways for your needs.

Sensational wardrobes for Avoiders

Avoiders want very little sensory input; this translates into limited wardrobe options. For others, limiting the wardrobe may seem depressing, but for the Avoiders, a limited wardrobe sets them free. If the wardrobe items don't overload the sensory systems, Avoiders have more resources available for other activities throughout the day.

The clothing industry has been responsive to feedback about how uncomfortable clothing tags feel by creating tagless clothing. Hanes led the way and other companies have followed to make clothing more comfortable for people. People who are Avoiders have many more choices when they can buy tagless wardrobe items and not worry about making holes in their clothing when they rip the uncomfortable tags out of them.

Avoiders who cannot tolerate input to the skin might love to be naked all the time; however, this isn't a good social strategy. Remembering the organizing and alerting categories of input to the skin, Avoiders really want to stay away from the alerting inputs (e.g. light tickly touch) and focus on the organizing inputs (firm, even pressure on the skin). The tight-fitting clothing needs to *fit*, and not bunch up anywhere; the bunching-up spots will drive the Avoider wild. So, clothing with some stretch so it molds to the exact surface of the body is the best choice. Avoiders who cannot tolerate visual input will want to wear monochromatic color schemes, and Avoiders who struggle with sound will prefer rubber-soled shoes and sparse jewelry (so it doesn't make sounds when you move).

Listen to how Randolph describes his choices:

> When I am shopping for clothing, I feel my way through the clothing department to find bulletproof, beefy fabric. T-shirts have to be thick dense, heavy. I hate dress t-shirts because they are too thin, so they have to be thick; I like the microfiber t-shirts, as they have weight and feel buttery on my skin. My socks have to be really dense, firm, and thick, like hiking socks, but cannot be woolly with hairs and nubs in the weaving. I am also very picky about my shoes. They have to feel right with my socks and skin. With my thick socks, I need shoes that are stout and heavy. That is why I think that wingtips are the perfect shoe. The sole is dense, the heel is thick, even the top is heavy over my foot. They even have nails in them to make them heavier. I look for them at estate sales because the older ones are heavier than newer ones. I even re-dyed my high school wingtips from brown to black so I could keep them. I have never understood how someone could wear two different shoes to work; a co-worker has done this. Of course, I would never get to work with two different shoes on because it would bug me way before I got there!

The Avoider's style is predictable

The Avoider's style is predictable. Avoiders will find clothing items that they like and will stick to them. They will wear preferred items until they are past worn out, and be reluctant to get new things. Avoiders may even purchase more than one of the same item; if they find jeans they really like, they will want to have back-up pairs so they don't have to contend with finding another pair that meets their needs. Style is likely to be clean and classic; Avoiders cannot tolerate additional sensory input and trendy styles often have adornments on them. Extra cuffs, collars, pockets, or bands on clothing create additional visual interest, but they also add stitching to the clothing that would be noticeable to an Avoider. Extra stitching can rub on the skin and be overwhelming to Avoiders, even though others wouldn't notice this additional feature.

Avoiders will select wardrobe items with a very narrow range of colors, smooth, even fabrics, and few if any accessories. Avoiders want their clothing to be easy to disregard; if Avoiders are noticing their clothing, they will be more easily overwhelmed by other things in their day.

Undergarments are critical to comfort and satisfaction. For Avoiders, this means that undergarments must provide as little input as possible. Tags are completely unacceptable, as are thin bands with elastic. Thin bands of elastic cut into the skin, and therefore provide intense sensory input. Soft fabric, even texture (with *no* nubs, not even tiny nubs in fabric from the threads being knotted) is helpful. Some Avoiders will prefer undergarments that are evenly close to the skin (e.g. boxer briefs, undershirts with Lycra), while other Avoiders will prefer soft fabric that fits loosely enough that the undergarment will cling to the outer clothing rather than the body. These choices can affect your leisure and exercise routines as well.

Ralph tells how it affects his running:

> I am a serious runner, and so there is some social pressure to wear just the right clothing. The problem is I hate the feeling of those light nylon running shorts, so I wear leggings underneath my running shorts to keep the running shorts from bugging me. I took a lot of ribbing at first, but this died away a lot faster than the feeling of those shorts!

General tips for a sensational Avoider wardrobe
Clothing:

  o predictable combinations

   o same basic components all the time.

Fabrics:

   o smooth even surfaces

   o monochromatic color schemes.

Accessories:

   o sparse or none.

Undergarments:

   o even textures

   o form-fitting with no tight places.

Tips for creating a sensational Avoider wardrobe

   o Select smooth, sleek fabrics with very little texture.

   o Find one pair of earrings that suits all outfits.

   o Get time from other devices to keep from having to use a watch.

   o Find one brand for socks and underwear and stock up.

   o Use no-scent products for cleaning clothing.

   o Wash new clothing before wearing the first time to remove starch/fragrances.

Sensational wardrobes for Sensors

Sensors will be very picky about shopping for their wardrobes. They will scour racks feeling all the clothes, inspect clothing items for details (e.g. fasteners, stitching), and will reject many choices. Sensors will tell you exactly what they can and cannot manage related to shoe shape, fabrics, waistbands, fasteners, the length of skirts, pants, shirts and jackets, and the weight of the clothing items. Sensors want their clothing to stay put, and will be intolerant of swishy, moving items. Sensors will wear minimum jewelry, won't like layering, and will likely have only one brand of socks and other underwear that is acceptable. They will also be very vocal about companies that discontinue their personal favorites.

The Sensor's style is very precise

The Sensor's style is very precise: they will identify a style of clothing that is comfortable, and create their wardrobe to portray this style all the time. Sensors will select smooth, sleek options that are very low on the "fussy" scale. Sensors will have a smaller wardrobe of preferred items, and will wear these preferred items frequently. They will be like Avoiders in their lack of interest in adornments; adornments provide more sensory opportunities, and this can easily overwhelm Sensors. Others won't understand the Sensor's objections to simple things, like a lapel pin, arguing that it's "no big deal"; the addition of a lapel pin adds weight, something to catch visual attention, and the backs poke into one's clothing just a little. That little amount of poking could drive a Sensor crazy all day long.

Sensors will select wardrobe items with particular colors, textures, and fabrics to meet their particular needs. Sensors will select fabrics that are light, almost non-existent, so as not to compete with other activities throughout the day. Fabrics will need to have smooth surfaces; textures like linen may have nubs on them that will be noticeable to the Sensor's skin. Processing chemicals that manufacturers use to prepare clothing for sale will also be negative features for Sensors. If a Sensor notices visual input, then clothing will be solid colors, with very little if any stripes, plaids, or patterns. Sensors are also likely to select a color palate for the entire wardrobe (e.g. black and khaki, or all pastels). The other advantage of smooth fabrics is that they make very little noise as the person moves in them. Sensors will also be very particular about cleaning their clothing, because the fragrance of soaps, dry cleaning, and other products will be very easy to detect.

Betty has a dilemma with her sensitivity to textures on her skin and the secret codes of dress in her industry. During the colder months, the women's dress code includes suits with turtleneck sweaters. She wants to look the part, so she purchases some well-fitting turtleneck sweaters. She can manage everything but the turtleneck part of the sweater, which bugs her all day long. She stuck panty liners to the inside of the neck area, so the softness of the liner would touch her skin; the firmness didn't bother her, just the texture, so she was good to go for the day. When clothing had tags sewn in so firmly that she couldn't remove them safely without harming the garment, she stuck a piece of moleskin over the tag too. Who knew her secrets to success at work?

Accessories for the Sensor are likely to be small, light, and sparse. Sensors will feel anything on their bodies, so accessories have to be as unobtrusive as possible. In fact, Sensors may wish to have no accessories (e.g. no tie, no earrings) but recognize the expectation in particular situations, and so hunt to find the least obtrusive options for them.

Ursula works in a high fashion retail store, so looking the part matters. As a Sensor, this has been challenging at times. I met her in her store, and as we chatted, the ideas about sensory patterns seeped into the conversation (imagine that!). For all intents and purposes, Ursula seemed like a Sensor, but she was wearing very funky, wild shoes, with a flower design and fur around the edges of the shoes. So I had to ask her about this because the shoes seemed like ones that a Seeker would wear. She replied:

> Oh I do love how these shoes look! But you are right, I couldn't bear to wear them without hosiery. They would have to drop me off at the clinic before lunch!

How clever of Ursula! She figured out how to mediate her Seeker tendencies for visual input (the shoes look great!) with her Sensor tendencies for touch (using hosiery to keep the feathers from touching her skin).

Undergarments are critical to your comfort and satisfaction with your wardrobe. For Sensors, this means that undergarments must not be noticeable throughout the day. Everything must stay in place without binding anywhere. Sensors will notice even small shifts in undergarments, so pieces must have just the right amount of "cling" and softness. It usually takes experimentation to get the right amount of firmness against the skin without being too tight. When things are too tight, moving makes the fabric clump around the bending areas. However, when items are too loose, movements cause the undergarment to brush against the skin lightly, causing a "tickling" feeling (the alerting system), and this can also be noticeable and therefore irritating for Sensors.

Consider the journey that Bill had to take to find the right underwear:

> Boy, do I have issues with clothing! Let's start with the underwear. I wore briefs for years, and was uncomfortable because they are too tight at the waist. I have tried boxer briefs, and I liked them better because they hug my skin, but they also have seams that run down my bottom

on both sides and this drives me crazy; I can feel those seams all day long. I am sure you can guess that I ended up with boxers, but that wasn't that easy either. The first ones I tried were thin, polished cotton, and these were very distressing because they were so thin that they moved around on me. Now I wear thicker flannel or knit boxers, and these are more satisfying because they stay put all day.

General tips for a sensational Sensor wardrobe

Clothing:

- precise styles
- personal favorites without deviation.

Fabrics:

- smooth, soft
- low texture.

Accessories:

- clean, small, sleek
- light in weight.

Undergarments:

- just the right fit
- no bunching or tickling.

Tips for creating a sensational Sensor wardrobe

- Stick to a style that is comfortable for you.
- Select a few reliable and small accessories.
- Select fabrics with smooth texture.
- Select lightweight items.
- Examine clothing seams to ensure they are flat and smooth.
- Identify perfect-fitting undergarments and stick with them.

Sensational wardrobes for Bystanders

Bystanders will have an easy time with dressing; they will not notice the details that Sensors and Avoiders detect throughout the day. Bystanders may solicit others to help with wardrobe planning because they don't attend to the shifts in fashion or realize the wardrobe expectations of particular situations. The challenge comes when Bystanders need to design a particular image. Since Bystanders don't notice sensory input the way others do, their clothing can be twisted on their bodies, buttoned unevenly, or even mismatched. Bystanders do better with easy-to-match, easy-to-wear clothing because this reduces the possibility of looking disheveled. It will also be helpful to have easy-to-clean clothing; since they may miss cues around them, they may step into puddles, spill things, or dribble onto their clothes. The good news is that Bystanders are also easy-going, so these events will not upset them at all.

The Bystander's style is easy-going

The Bystander's style is likely to be easy-going and casual. They will be more broad-minded about the fit of clothing; a little tighter or looser won't be noticeable nor will it matter. Bystanders may have "outfits" in their wardrobe so they can make sure to get a look put together without having to remember what goes together. For example, a man will have one or two ties for each shirt; a woman will have a skirt or trousers matching one pair of shoes, and then have selected tops for each set. Bystanders will do well with brands that match tops and bottoms as a set.

Mai took a new job as a sales rep for the entire mid-section of the country. She knew that she would have to look sharp as she traveled to meet distributors and retailers. Pulling her wardrobe together was challenging for Mai; she had a reputation in college for being funky, and on bad days, a little off the mark with regard to style. She just couldn't get all excited about all those details, like layering (except if it was really cold), mixing and matching accessories, and wearing "complementary" shoes:

> [Sigh!] People in the dorm would say I shouldn't match my shoe color to my outfit exactly, but that they should "go with" my clothes. What the heck does that mean?

She decided to go to a favorite store and buy whole outfits they had already put together, and then take those outfits directly to the shoe store and have the sales people select shoes for her. Mai is a Bystander who has come up with a great strategy for managing her need to have a put-together look for her new job.

Bystanders select similar wardrobe items over and over. They won't spend energy worrying about the details of getting an outfit put together, so staying with tried and true items works for them. Their easy-going style reflects the fact that wardrobe details that others find so important just don't matter to them. They may also find an entire outfit on the mannequin in a store, and purchase all the items in that outfit to create a trendy look without having to pay attention to how to create the look for themselves.

Bystanders may or may not use accessories. There may be days that they think about adding accessories, and other days when accessories are left at home. They are more likely to include accessories in their wardrobe when they have been selected for a particular outfit, because the outfit provides a reminder to put the accessories on. For example, a shirt with French cuffs provides a cue for getting cufflinks out. A woman might leave a brooch on a jacket so it is there when she puts that jacket on.

Undergarments are also easier for Bystanders. They will not be sensitive to the bands, length, and fit of items, so many styles of undergarments will be acceptable for them. Because the details are not important, Bystanders may select undergarment brands and styles that they wore growing up; they won't feel any need to make adjustments. The cool thing is that unlike other people, undergarments will not interfere with the Bystander's day; anything goes.

Michael is a middle-aged man who is a Bystander with his wardrobe. After his parents visited for a weekend, his wife noticed that Michael's briefs were sagging as he was getting ready for work on Monday morning. He got out the door before she could ask him about it. When sorting the laundry the next week, Beth noticed that they had a pair of Michael's dad's briefs, which were two sizes larger than Michael's. He and his wife had a laugh at Michael's flexibility in wearing briefs that weren't even his size. His wife Beth, who is a Sensor, commented that she would have felt the difference in the fabric just pulling the item out of the laundry basket, and wouldn't have even dressed in them. Beth was somewhat jealous that Michael could wear the wrong size all day without being bothered by it. She told Michael how her whole day could be disrupted if a thread gets loose on her underwear.

General tips for a sensational Bystander wardrobe

Clothing:

- ○ easy-going
- ○ preplanned outfits.

Fabrics:

- ○ all types of fabrics will be OK.

Accessories:

- ○ not mandatory
- ○ best when paired with particular outfits.

Undergarments:

- ○ likely to retain styles throughout life
- ○ details are not important.

Tips for creating a sensational Bystander wardrobe

- ○ Purchase an outfit that is illustrated on the mannequin in a store so that a trendy style is effortless.
- ○ Identify items that form an outfit in your closet.
- ○ Keep accessories with particular clothing items.
- ○ Shop with a Seeker friend.

9

Your Home Is your Castle: Creating Living Spaces that Meet Your Sensory Needs

In this chapter, you will discover how to make your living spaces perfect for your sensory needs. The chapter begins with the story of Aden, who created a haven for himself, and then his brother begins to share his home. The chapter continues with a discussion of the important factors in creating sensational living spaces, that is, location within a community, buildings, and floor plans, and decorating with the senses in mind. Then there is a discussion of optimal living spaces for people with each of the four sensory patterns. In the final section of the chapter, there is a discussion about how to negotiate shared living spaces with the senses in mind.

Opening story

It's my sacred space, so leave it alone!

Aden had worked hard to purchase his home. He picked it because it was at the end of the street, and so there was very little traffic to contend with. He designed the inside to be sleek and clean. Cabinets had smooth fronts, with very little hardware. Aden liked everything put away, and he had a specific place for all his belongings. His furniture was firm and arranged symmetrically in the room. Aden installed dimmers on all the light switches so he could control the brightness in each room. He added an extra large venting system to the kitchen to remove smells from cooking. He loved his home, and found solace there.

When Aden's brother finished college, he got a job in Aden's town, and moved in with Aden for a while until he could find a place of his own. Richard moved into the basement so he and Aden could have their own spaces.

Richard was a little more casual than Aden. Richard picked up his clothing from the floor of his bedroom and bathroom when it was time to do the laundry. He turned on the stereo as soon as he got home and sometimes sang along. He loved to cook, so he offered to do the cooking for Aden while he was staying there. By the time Aden got home, the aroma of dinner and the sound of the stereo filled the air. Richard was happy to see his brother, and to be helping by making dinner:

> "Hey dude, could we turn the tunes down? I need some quiet when I get home." (Aden)

> "The music motivates me, and I am making a rocking dinner for us." (Richard)

> "So use your MP3 player then; I can't hear myself think." (Aden)

Richard tried to clean up after dinner, but Aden insisted on clean-up duty. He feared that Richard would not clean to his liking, and wanted his utensils and dishes put in the right place. Richard frequently left his morning dishes in the sink, so Aden knew that clean-up needed his personal attention.

Aden is an Avoider in his living spaces. He wants the smallest amount of sensory input in his home. He wants low light (keeping the shades down, dimmer switches), a small number of visual distractions (very few decorations, flat fronts on cabinets, everything put away), no extra sounds (asking his brother to use his earphones) and no lingering odors (extra large vent in kitchen). When his brother comes to stay, he places him in a separate space so that Richard's personal clutter won't be bothersome.

Aden has developed some great strategies for managing his living space to keep sensory input to a minimum. These strategies keep him from getting overwhelmed, and enable him to regroup. His brother Richard had the potential to disrupt Aden's safe space; luckily, Aden understood enough about what he needed to ask Richard to change, and to compartmentalize where Richard spent time.

Introduction

Your living space is sacred. This space serves as a grounding place, sometimes as a retreat from the hectic outside world, sometimes as a place to re-energize. When you understand your sensory processing preferences, you can use this knowledge to make your living spaces *exactly* how your senses need the space to be.

What words would you use to describe your own or someone else's living space? When a person has a smaller number of carefully selected decorative items, we might call it "minimalist" or "sleek." We might also call that same living space cold or stark. Another home might be described as warm, cozy and inviting, or dense, full, and cluttered. Differences in sensory processing preferences contribute to how you select, organize, and accessorize your own living spaces, and how you react to other people's living spaces.

Your living space is central to your ability to function every day. When your living spaces are just the way your senses need them to be, you feel powerful and organized. Yet, everyone has experienced times when living spaces were unsettling. Perhaps you lived with room-mates who had a different idea about what a clean apartment was, or perhaps early in your professional life you had second-hand furniture that provided seating, rest, and storage, but wasn't exactly your "style." Even in loving relationships, partners can have very strong reactions when moving in together and making decisions about "yours," "mine," and "ours." Many of these negotiations are rooted in your sensory preferences.

Paul and Eliana were blending their single lives as they planned to move in together. They had too much furniture, so had to negotiate about what to keep. Eliana was completely unwilling to part with the couch she had saved for; it was a wonderfully rich brocade fabric that made Eliana feel regal. For Paul, this couch was a nightmare:

I agree with Eliana that this is a beautiful couch. It has great style and the colors are perfect for our home. But I have to have armor on to sit on the darn thing. Without extra layers of clothing, I can feel the fibers poking through my clothing to irritate my skin. I shouldn't have to "suit up" to sit on my couch.

The situation was challenging. It seemed insolvable until one day in desperation, Paul sank into his favorite, but very worn leather chair:

Sitting in this chair is like being the baseball in a well-worn glove. It just melts into your skin and hugs you.

Eliana wasn't so taken by Paul's leather chair, and preferred a matching chair. What turned the tide was Paul's comment that he loved looking at Eliana's couch, and that he could do this from his leather chair without having to sit on the couch. He reminded Eliana that she didn't like being around him when he was cranky. They settled on the leather chair and the new couch.

Paul has very narrow tolerances for touch input; the familiar leather chair met his needs, and the newer, textured couch wasn't tolerable. He is an Avoider in this situation, and needs to have options for sitting that he can tolerate so he can focus on their conversation, or the TV show, or guests.

Your individual sensory nature contributes to what makes you feel comfortable at home. Sensors and Avoiders are more likely to prefer living spaces with carefully selected items, specific kinds of lighting, and furniture with exactly the "right" amount of support and comfort. Seekers are more likely to have a menagerie of items in each room. Bystanders are comfortable in many types of living spaces, since they tend not to notice things.

As we have discussed in other chapters, the exact nature of these decisions will also depend on which sensations are most important to each person. For example, a person may enjoy visual input and have lots of art around the home, but be sensitive to auditory input and want the stereo very low or even turned off.

Living spaces have to be situated within the community itself (address), the structures have characteristics (buildings), the living spaces have particular qualities (floor plan), and each space must be adorned (room decorating) to suit the person(s) living in that space.

Here are some ideas to get you started. Your sensory patterns within your living spaces might show up in these ways.

You are a Seeker in living spaces if you:

○ have lots of decorations

○ move the furniture around more than once a year

○ have background sound going all the time (e.g. TV, stereo)

○ use scented air fresheners

○ choose furniture with textures

○ have brightly lit rooms.

You are a Bystander in your living spaces if you:

○ miss a new decorative item your room-mate purchased

○ recognizes that rooms are cluttered but hadn't noticed until someone pointed it out

○ feel clumsy for a while when things are rearranged

○ are easy-going about background music in the home.

You are an Avoider in living spaces if you:

○ have sparse decorations

○ keep shades down

○ want a quiet space away from the family

○ have a "retreat" area

○ close doors when in a room

○ use headphones without any music to increase the quiet

○ use only unscented cleaning products.

You are a Sensor in your living spaces if you:

○ are very particular about placement of furniture and decorations

○ frequently readjust and rearrange items to straighten them

○ want very low volume in TV and stereo

○ take a long time to select new furniture and decorations

○ have a precise idea about where everything "belongs."

Location in the community

The first consideration for living spaces is where in the community you will live. You consider location in a community related to price, availability, neighborhoods, schools, transportation routes, or access to preferred activities (e.g. grocery stores, movie theaters, medical services). These considerations and others (e.g. urban, suburban, country) are all important factors in ending up in a satisfying location. With the additional consideration of your sensory processing needs, you can refine your community selection, and meet your sensory needs as well.

Type of housing

When you think about living spaces, the type of housing is also a consideration. The structure of a building, whether it is collective housing (such as a duplex or apartment building) or single dwelling, supports particular sensory experiences. For example, a home that has all windows ceiling to floor on one side of it to afford a view provides a very different sensory environment from a row house that only has windows in the front and back due to the proximity of other houses next door. All of us are attracted to certain types of buildings, and do not consider other types. Avoiders may be more attracted to homes with only a few windows or end-of-hall apartments, while Seekers may be more attracted to unusual and interesting architecture and placement in a property. If you have had housing that felt unsettling to you, it may have been a bad match for your sensory needs.

The style of the building, entrances, placement on property, landscaping, and building materials all reflect different sensory preferences. Sparse design features are more attractive to Sensors and Avoiders; busy design features are more useful for Bystanders and Seekers.

Characteristics of the living space

Now we are inside the living space. The first major consideration within living spaces is the layout and organization of the space. Many styles are available for this internal organization, and particular styles will be best suited to people with different sensory patterns. Characteristics to consider are the floor plan, height of ceilings, and placement of hallways and stairs. Your sensory processing preferences may underlie your attractions to and distaste for particular floor plans because they have the potential to meet your needs.

Decorating your home

Another factor to consider inside living spaces is the accessories, adornments, or decorations you use to make the space your own. This personalization process can be highly effective to meet your sensory needs. For example, you may need to live in a particular part of town, or in a specific building because of work convenience or cost, even though those locations are busier (or more isolated) than you would prefer to meet your sensory needs. Insulated window coverings can reduce the impact of bright light or sounds (for Sensors or Avoiders); sheer window coverings can invite light and sounds in while maintaining privacy. You have the most control over your accessories and decorations, and so can make excellent choices that meet your sensory needs.

Location in the community, arrangement and decor of spaces all contain opportunities for meeting your sensory needs. Let's consider what strategies people with each sensory pattern might use within their living spaces.

Living spaces for Seekers

Seekers will want to look for community locations that are busy, with unusual traffic patterns of roads/entrances. You might want to be in a location that has heavy traffic, and lots of activity throughout the day, or near where the community gathers for special events (e.g. parade or marathon routes, parks with public events). With a busier community location, you will have naturally occurring opportunities to get the information/input you need to stay engaged throughout the day/week. If you are interested in apartment or condo living, select a busier part of the building (e.g. near the mailboxes or fitness center). If you are interested in single family homes, select a location on a busier street, or near the entrance to a neighborhood.

Derek lived in a second floor apartment that faced a busy street. He gave notice to the landlady when he wanted to move to a quieter location. Derek told the landlady she might want to tell applicants about the busy street and resulting traffic and crowd noise. She seemed amused, and commented that some people enjoyed that activity and level of noise because it made them feel part of the city.

Derek is a Sensor who wants to have a quieter living space. A Seeker or Bystander would be fine in this apartment. Seekers would enjoy the bustle of the city; Bystanders might not notice all the activity unless they had guests who noticed and pointed it out.

Seekers feel more satisfied with housing that has unusual architectural designs, or that has more adornments, such as shutters, porches, or multiple roof lines. Interesting gardens that are dense and contain a variety of flowers (some fragrant), shrubs, and unusual entryways would also be attractive to Seekers. They provide the variety that enables Seekers to meet their high sensory needs more easily.

Seekers want a floor plan that has some interest to increase sensory input throughout the day. Seekers enjoy open living spaces that connect rooms without doors so you can frequently rearrange the space. High ceilings with fans, or spaces open to the second story, create opportunities to hear and smell and see what is going on in the home.

Seekers go wild with decorating, taking advantage of colors, textures, and arrangements

Seekers go wild with decorating! Take advantage of bright, contrasting color schemes and wall textures, including wallpapers and fabrics. Window dressings can be interesting while remaining open to let in light, sounds, and smells from the outside. Eclectic art can be displayed, providing interest in each room. Use a variety of fabrics and textures for furniture, blankets, pillows, or wall hangings. Flooring from room to room can also be varied with linoleum, area rugs, and carpeting.

Sena loves art. She has all types of art all over her home. She thinks every surface (including tables, counters, walls, doors) is an invitation to decorate. She has art hanging on every door, has clusters of art on every wall space, and uses shelves and tables to display collections of objects. Even workspaces have baskets full of pens, scissors, and paper in case someone gets an inspiration to create something.

Sena has parties for co-workers every few months. One of her co-workers, Lorie, loves Sena, but has to manage herself in Sena's home. She prefers to go to the spring, summer, and fall parties because she can go out on the deck to get a mental breather from the intensity of Sena's home.

As a Seeker, Sena is loading up her home with art and art supplies for everyone to enjoy. As an Avoider, Lorie has to get away from the intense sensory environment in order to interact with others at the party.

Ideas for Seekers in living spaces

Within the community:

- o Select the main street of town.

- o Live in complexes/neighborhoods with gathering places.

- o In an apartment building, live near the elevator where there is more activity.

Type of housing:

- o Select front of building locations.

- o Choose interesting/unusual home design.

- o Select unusual entrances.

- o Create perennial gardens that change throughout the season.

Floor plans:

- o Select open living spaces connecting rooms without doors to increase interactivity within the space.

- o Look for uneven placement of windows and doorways for movement and visual interest.

- o Look for high ceilings or open halls to second story so that more can be heard about what is going on.

- o Consider multiple levels separated by one to three steps.

Decorating:

- o Choose bright, contrasting color schemes to increase visual stimulation.

- o Select multiple kinds of art adorning the rooms.

- o Increase the multiple textures in rooms to create visual and tactile interest.

- o Include varied flooring to increase variability when moving around.

Bystanders in living spaces

Bystanders will do best in community locations that are busy, unusual, or interesting, just like the sensation-seekers. Bystanders do not work to include their sensory needs like Seekers do, however. Unpredictability is a strong factor for Bystanders because when a sensory event comes unexpectedly, Bystanders are more likely to detect it. It is easier to ignore or pass by sensory events that come in a predictable pattern.

Julian lives in the path of bus routes so he can get to places easily. However, he frequently misses the bus because there is so much activity at the route intersection that he misses his own bus:

> There just seems to be a rhythm at the bus stop that flows the same way every day. I get caught up in the rhythm and miss my bus.

However, when Julian is on his way to a sporting event, he takes more notice of the increased traffic because it is unusual:

> Taking the bus to a game is very different. People are in a frenzy, and I get bumped a lot, and hear people talking about the game, and people are wearing weird clothes too.

Julian needs the additional and unpredictable input of the game day to get the input he needs to stay focused on the task of getting somewhere. The routine of going to work from his home nearby is too predictable to be "detectable" to his sensory systems.

Bystanders are more easily satisfied than other groups, but Bystanders have to consider selecting housing types that will meet their thresholds so they can stay engaged with activities in their life. Therefore, Bystanders need to select housing that will capture attention. For example, Bystanders might select housing with entrances from several places (e.g. front door, garage, porch, or parking lot, elevator, and stairwell). Living in a home or building with perennial gardens means that they will change often, so this is also a good alternative.

Bystanders need housing layouts that are challenging. When the floor plan invites more movement, repositioning, or hearing things from room to room, there is a greater chance for Bystanders to keep their sensory systems activated, and therefore stay engaged in the routines of everyday life. Look for halls where the doorways do not line up, multilevel homes with a few steps up and down into living spaces, or apartments with archways or angled walls.

Bystanders profit from an eclectic and varied style of decorating

Bystanders profit from an eclectic and varied style of decorating. Place eye-catching items in each room, or add wind chimes or small fountains to add sound to the space. Room deodorizers can also add an aroma to a room, including spritzers of food aromas for the kitchen. Less efficient room arrangements can also be helpful.

Basel's partner Celeste is very creative with room design. She placed furniture in the room in unusual patterns so people would have to walk around the couch to sit down; this requires more attention as a person moves around the room. Celeste's internal motive (besides being interested in trying new things) is to keep Basel paying attention around the home. He is clumsy, and bumps into things if he isn't watching where he is going. She also placed timers on lighting, so it goes on and off at different times to increase Basel's alertness. About once every two months, she moves the wall decorations around as well.

Basel has a great partner in Celeste. She creates a changeable living space to keep Basel's attention. The changing visual and movement experiences keep his sensory systems active. This is critical for Bystanders.

Ideas for Bystanders in living spaces

Within the community:

- Select a location in the path of typical errands to provide reminders.
- Choose a space near landmarks to provide cues.
- Select housing near distinctive features of neighborhood.

Type of housing:

- Go for buildings with directional cues and signs as reminders.
- Select distinctive home designs.
- Look for homes with noticeable landscaping.
- Install automatic (movement-sensitive, dusk/dawn) lighting outside.

Floor plans:

o Look for unusual floor plans to provide variability in everyday routines.

o Go for plans with visual and sound access from one room to another to make it easier to know what is going on.

o Create open shelving so belongings are easier to notice.

o Change the flooring from room to room to increase attention when moving around.

o Install different lighting options throughout each room.

Decorating:

o Select a more variable, eclectic style to maintain interest.

o Include eye-catching items in rooms to attract attention.

o Opt for unusual arrangements and change them frequently.

o Select many varying textures in fabrics for visual and tactile input.

o Place timers on lighting and vary when different areas go on and off.

o Add night lights in halls and bathrooms.

o Place mirrors in several locations to provide variety in the view of each room.

Sensors in living spaces

Sensors look for community locations that are near, but not in the path of, community activities. Sensors need a community location that allows both "get away" options, and access to activities when personal resources are available to participate without being overwhelmed. When selecting a community location in a familiar town, consider familiar neighborhoods (e.g. know where the grocery stores are, how to get to places). When relocating, take some time to drive around within a neighborhood to look for signs of comfortable layouts. Compile a list of preferences/dislikes from a current location, and rate the new locations with these factors involved. Visit a location several times of day/week to determine the characteristics across the time periods.

Nick lived in a neighborhood that had a food processing plant close by. Once a week, it emitted fumes that smelled like the burnt, undesirable version of their product. Nick thought he had been very attentive when looking for his apartment. He wanted only shrubs around the building because they don't "stink" like flowers do. He asked for a back-of-building apartment to get away from the nearby fast food restaurants. Nick only found out about this emission after moving in on a year-long lease. He was very sensitive to smells, and so had to rearrange his work and school schedule to make sure he was not home when the plant emissions occurred.

Nick is a Sensor in living situations, particularly for smells. He was aware of his own sensitivity, and yet got stuck in a situation that was unpleasant anyway.

Sensors feel more comfortable with housing that has good insulation, clean/sparse lines in design, and more sculpted landscaping. Sensors prefer a predictable pattern of entry into the housing, including both the arrangement of walkways, and the landscaping around them. For example, shrubs and evergreens might be a better choice for the front of the housing because their image remains relatively stable over time, and they don't have a fragrance like flowers do (e.g. Nick, above). When the path and landscaping remain the same across seasons, it is one less issue to contend with when entering the residence.

Sensors prefer floor plans that are functional and efficient

Sensors are attracted to floor plans that are more functionally organized. Arrangements in which sections of the living space are dedicated to particular activities are desirable (e.g. the back hall is for the bedrooms; the far corner is for the desk/work area). Sensors also prefer rooms with uninterrupted wall spaces to provide continuity of the space (which is less distracting).

Sensors need to identify favorite color and art styles and stick with them for decorating the living space. Sensors enjoy designing a specific place to display a piece of art, so the artistic qualities are highlighted in the living space. Arrange furniture for ease and efficiency, making it easy for people to gather and to retreat. Focused lighting in functional locations can also be useful, to create a sense of intimacy and containment for the activity.

Beth has fond memories of her grandmother's couch:

I remember the feeling of being on that couch from when I was a little girl. It was covered in the most beautiful blue velvet, and I couldn't wait to put my skin up against the velvet. I felt like the couch was soothing me, it was so soft. I would lie on it and pet the surface over and over again until I fell asleep there.

Imagine Beth's delight when she heard that her parents had retrieved the couch from her grandmother's home when they moved her to an older adults, living community. She couldn't wait to get home and reminisce on the couch.

Beth was shocked when she arrived home and her parents proudly escorted her to the *newly upholstered* couch! Although the new fabric was beautiful, it was scratchy to Beth. She and her parents had to have a long talk about the couch that evening. Now they laugh that when Beth gets the couch, she will reupholster it in blue velvet.

Beth has very particular rules about what feels good on her skin, but she probably didn't communicate those details to her family in relation to grandma's couch. They saw what pleasure she got from the couch, and thought it was the *couch* that mattered. Her parents wanted to get the treasure all cleaned up for Beth, never realizing that the velvet was what mattered to Beth. Sensors like Beth don't always know why they are so particular until they encounter the contrast between what is acceptable and what is unacceptable to them.

Ideas for Sensors in living spaces

Within the community:

- Select a quiet street close to activity to manage amount of input.
- Choose a familiar neighborhood so there are less surprises.
- Live near friends and family that understand you.

Type of housing:

- Select buildings with good insulation to reduce sounds and temperature shifts.
- Choose clean/sparse lines in design to reduce distractibility.
- Install sculpted landscaping to reduce distractibility.

○ Select symmetrical designs.

○ Look for easy access in and out of building.

Floor plans:

○ Identify zoned floor plans, with functions grouped together to increase focus.

○ Look for expansive, uninterrupted wall spaces in each room to create a calm, visual space.

Decorating:

○ Stick with favorite colors in the same color family (e.g. same tones in the colors, or shades of the same color).

○ Create specific locations for displaying a favorite piece of art to focus visual interest in one place.

○ Organize accessories to create clear arrangement for particular functions in the space (e.g. work zone).

○ Design clear and focused lighting strategies.

Avoiders in living spaces

Avoiders look for community locations that are more isolated and remote from community activity. Dead-end streets, basement apartments, apartments at the end of the hall, and more rural locations are all desirable community locations for Avoiders. Since sensory input overwhelms Avoiders more easily, it is critical that community locations provide a place for resting and regrouping. When the community location provides too much sensory input, Avoiders are on alert when rest is needed. There are enough times during the day that are challenging; living spaces need to be the most compatible with Avoiders' sensory needs.

> Avoiders prefer more contained
> spaces that provide getaways

Avoiders feel comfortable in more contained spaces that afford separateness. Quieter back entrances or entrance through a closed garage are better choices. Avoiders select housing with fewer windows, or which provide areas without windows to reduce light, sound, and smells that come into the residence. They prefer to select housing with plainer facades and entry paths, and yards with getaway places in them that are separated from the rest of the outside space.

Amir was renovating his home. He was very particular about how he wanted the changes to be made. His home is built into the side of a hill, so the entire back of the house is in contact with the earth:

> I love my house being in contact with the earth. This way we cannot have windows on the whole back and part of the sides of the house. It's not that I hate the light, in fact I *love* the light coming in to warm the house. But windows also let in sounds from the street, so it is good that we have only a few windows in the front of the house. I do have some skylights to let in the light. Anyway, we get most of the rehab finished, and we need a garage door opener. I research and find out that there is a *silent* garage door opener! I am thrilled, and even though it costs US$1000, I will pay any price to keep that horrible sound from intruding on my haven. You know the sound: metal on metal, grinding, and churning. So they install it, and *I can still hear it!* Now I am determined; just the idea that I *could* have quiet means I can't stop now. So I take the whole thing down, disassemble it, and add rubber gaskets, and reinstall it. *Finally*, the peace we deserve.

What is interesting about this story is that for many people, the sound of the garage door opener is consoling and organizing. We hear it and know that our family members are home. We hear it and know that our children have gotten out of the garage successfully. We hear it and know that our home is secure for the night. We use the sound of the garage door opener to organize part of our days. But for Amir, an Avoider, the sound is very disruptive to his peace of mind.

Avoiders search for self-contained spaces in the floor plan. When rooms are more self-contained, it is easier to control the amount and type of sensory information available at any given time. Having a room without windows, or within which the window light, breeze, and sound can be controlled, will also be desirable features. Other general characteristics for Avoiders are lower ceilings, halls with rooms that can be closed off, and solid doors to block out external activity.

Avoiders create a sparser decorating scheme, with few selected items to accent the living space. Furniture serves not only its usual function, but also as barriers to reduce and define each space specifically within the living areas. Create spaces for being alone; when in a family, those spaces can be a corner in a larger space so other family can still see everyone. For example, you can place a reading chair in a corner behind other furniture, in a space that is out of the traffic flow of the living space. Avoiders prefer color schemas within one color grouping (e.g. different shades of taupe).

Ideas for Avoiders in living spaces

Within the community:

- Select buildings at the end of streets to reduce ambient noise and activity.

- Select apartments in the interior of the building to protect from external noise and activity.

- Consider country/rural locations to reduce density of people, sounds, movement, and so on.

- Consider a basement apartment if there is more insulation; check for noise in floors above before selecting this option.

Type of housing:

- Select straightforward entrances to get in and out easily.

- Look for easy access to parking to reduce complexity at beginning and end of work day.

- Consider housing with limited windows.

- Look for smooth external building materials to minimize visual façade.

- Add soundproofing building materials to protect spaces.

Floor plans:

- Go for self-contained spaces in floor plan to serve as getaways.

- Look for at least one room without windows.

- Select lower ceilings to contain spaces.

- Check doors in home, preferring solid doors.

- Have a room situated off hallway with doors that can be closed to create a getaway place.

Decorating:

- Choose sparse furniture and accessory designs.

- Select homogeneous color schemas.

- Create self-contained spaces within rooms.

- Arrange furniture to create quiet/separate corners for "being alone," for example, a chair in a corner separate from rest of room space.

Selecting and designing living spaces for room-mates and family groups

Most of us must negotiate our selected community location with other people that we will be living with. The chances are, in these situations, that the people involved will have different sensory processing preferences. Although this might seem impossible, or insurmountable, there are some strategies that are useful to make family life effective for all members.

For example, if one member is an Avoider and another member is a Seeker, a moderately busy community location affords the Seeker access to outside activities. Look for a home with solid doors, shades, and a more private room or section of the home so the Avoider can reduce sensory input once inside.

For a family with a Seeker and a Sensor, select a location on the edge of a neighborhood to provide both a quieter location and easy access. Then select a color scheme inside that is consistent with the Sensor's preferences, and add art within the color scheme that the Seeker enjoys. The Seeker could also have pens, pads, deck of cards, table games, books, toys, or an MP3 player in nearby drawers to be used when needed to increase sensory input for the Seeker.

Chapters 5 and 6 contain other suggestions for combining different sensory patterns successfully.

10

Work Is Life Too: Knowing Sensory Patterns at Work Helps You Succeed

Many of us spend a lot of time at work. Therefore, this life setting is also a place for understanding sensory patterns. As with all the topics in this book, sensory patterns are not the only explanation for what happens; sensory knowledge provides another helpful tool for making sure work is as productive and satisfying as possible.

Opening story

If people would just leave me alone, I could get my work done

Jacob is the manager of a small business. He is very happy with the company and overall loves his work, but all the intrusions throughout the day wear him down. Being a small company, everyone feels comfortable using each other's spaces and supplies, and to interrupt with questions whenever they pop up. Although this creates a sense of ownership and loyalty for the employees, it creates a sense of chaos for Jacob.

Jacob feels completely worn out at the end of the day with all the intrusions. After everyone leaves, he stays for another 45 minutes to get everything back in its proper place, and reset some order into his work areas. He tries to remain positive, but he is incredulous about how people can work in this business for years and not recognize how the office is supposed to be organized. Tidying up at the end of the day makes Jacob feel better, but he has another motive too:

> I figure if I show people the right way for the office to be organized, they will pick up these ideas and start putting things back where they belong. I have to admit that it doesn't seem to help, and I am wondering whether people have started to expect that I will clean up, so they don't have to.

There are certain staff that frustrate Jacob more than others. Two people in particular seem to disrupt the work areas to the point that Jacob has to stop working:

> Peggy and Don come into the work areas like bats out of hell. They enter talking on their cell phones, laughing, carrying bags that they plop down, and all the stuff slides out (because they haven't packed the bags properly). They don't even notice that they are upsetting things, and continue to act cheery as they take over the whole space. I have to admit that I feel irritated sometimes, but they don't seem to notice when I stick to business duties. I know it is good that they are positive since they are our marketing and sales people, but I wish they would check that jubilant attitude at the door. We have a business to run in here!

Jacob has a lot of responsibilities for this work setting flowing smoothly. We must never minimize these aspects of work when considering sensory needs along with the need to continue to work productively. And there are certainly many reasons for situations like those described above to occur. Peggy and Don could just be rude; Jacob could be a little unsure of himself, which could lead to feeling the need to exercise some control where he can. However, if we look at this situation from a sensory patterns point of view, there are also some possibilities about what is driving these behaviors. By considering the sensory patterns, we open up some possibilities about how to change the work setting to be more helpful to everyone.

Let's consider Jacob's sensory patterns and needs first. He feels the need to have order. At first, it seems that the visual environment is most troubling, with things strewn around and "not in their place." But then we also see that the auditory and movement disruptions from Peggy and Don are upsetting as well. His high detection of disorder and "chaos" and his personal challenge to keep everything in its place suggests that Jacob has a low tolerance for unexpected sensory input. So, is he a Sensor or an Avoider? Both these patterns have high detection and low tolerance for sensory input.

If Jacob were an Avoider, I suspect that he would have another job by now. He would have moved to a job that allowed him to be more isolated from others and all the random activity that occurs in this small business. It is more likely that Jacob is a Sensor; he notices everything very quickly and gets his fill, but he hangs in there, trying to get control over the situation whenever possible. He gets irritated sometimes, probably when his system has had enough sensory input and he doesn't find easy ways to get control over the situation to reduce the sensory onslaught. Peggy and Don are overwhelming to Jacob because they provide so much input so quickly. Even with the overall chaos, Jacob does better when he can regain control over the situation for himself, for example, when he cleans up at the end of the day. This is also a quieter time with less noise and less movement around him, so his sensory systems can take a breath and settle down before going home.

And then we have Peggy and Don to think of. We don't know a lot about them from this short story, but we do know that they are balls of energy and that they stir things up when they come into the work area. If we assume that they are kind, considerate people, then we can look at their behaviors from a sensory point of view. They are creating a lot of sensory input for themselves and others as they enter the work areas. They seem happy about what they are doing, and are not distressed. These traits lead us to think about people with high thresholds for sensory input, so are they Bystanders or Seekers?

We don't really know enough about them to decide between Bystanders and Seekers, so let's consider what would lead us in each direction. If Peggy or Don were Bystanders, then we might discover that they missed an appointment, wouldn't notice that their bags had spilled all over the floor (and might walk on their materials!), or wouldn't notice Jacob's building irritation. Remember, we are seeing the situation from Jacob's point of view; coming in like "bats out of hell" could be someone stumbling in (which would be a Bystander's entrance) or someone bursting in (which would be a Seeker's entrance). As Seekers, Peggy or Don would be more likely to have some new and unusual ideas for marketing, would have some interesting wardrobe selections, or would be singing the song from their car radio.

So what can we do for these conscientious but challenging work partners? There are many possibilities. Since Jacob manages the business, he could set up designated spaces for different aspects of the work, so people would have places to accomplish certain tasks. Jacob could purchase multiple copies of materials and tools that people use a lot in the business, so Jacob could keep his materials and tools organized in his personal workspace, while still making things available to other workers in another designated work area. This strategy would give Jacob a sense of order and control over some of his sensory needs, which can provide more "room" for dealing with the natural chaos of other people moving about. Perhaps there are options for entry that could be reorganized so staff like Peggy and Don could enter and put their things down in a less conspicuous location, and then engage with the rest of the staff without all their things in tow.

Introduction

We spend as much or more of our time at work than in any other activity of our lives, so it is really important to understand how our sensory patterns can affect us at work. There is an interesting constellation of forces that come to bear on our work, including the requirements of the job, the way work is organized and scheduled, the people we work with, the setting of our work, and our personal resources that enable us to be productive in our work. Our personal sensory patterns affect our decisions in each of these categories. Table 6 summarizes how our sensory patterns affect each of these aspects of our work.

> By considering sensory patterns,
> we open up possibilities about how to change
> the work setting to be more helpful to everyone

Table 6: Optimal work features for each sensory pattern

	Seekers	Bystanders	Avoiders	Sensors
Requirements of the job	○ Expectations of creative problem-solving ○ Multiple projects at same time	○ Expectations of productivity with deadlines laid out ○ Flexibility about how jobs are completed	○ Expectations of productivity within a specified routine	○ Expectations of precision in work projects ○ Control over job projects
Way work is organized and scheduled	○ Flexible schedule to allow for spontaneous opportunities and ideas	○ Expectations and timelines clear, blocks of time organized for work completion	○ Very structured, with a specified schedule and timelines	○ Structured, with advanced warning of changes
People we work with	○ Other Seekers/Bystanders for creative problem-solving ○ Sensors/Avoiders for keeping Seeker on deadlines and managing easily overlooked details	○ Avoiders/Sensors to provide structure for job tasks ○ Other Seekers to provide extra stimulation during work	○ Other Avoiders to complete independent work ○ Presence of Seekers at a distance for unusual work solutions	○ Bystanders because they will be flexible with the precision needs Sensors have
Settings of work	○ Busy, noisy, bustling, casual, movable furniture	○ In travel paths so there are interruptions ○ Open organization	○ Quiet, structured, isolated	○ Organized, clean, exclusively their own
Personal resources for work	○ Energetic and creative ○ Open to considering a wide range of possibilities	○ Easy-going and flexible	○ Organized and definite	○ Particular and detail-oriented
Preferred communication strategies	○ Meetings with flexible agenda	○ Meetings in another location	○ E-mail with time to respond ○ Time to research issues	○ Text messaging ○ Brief bullet points ○ Prepare ahead

Work settings have to be managed just like other settings. Just as in families at home, there will be people with various sensory patterns in the workplace, and we each have to negotiate ways to get the work accomplished and meet everyone's sensory needs too. Before understanding sensory patterns, we are more likely to get irritated by the quirky things our co-workers do; with sensory knowledge, we can be proactive, and even amused by our own and others' behaviors.

You are a Seeker at work if you:

o like busy work environments

o are flexible and creative about project possibilities

o work on multiple projects at the same time.

You are an Avoider at work if you:

o want a specific routine for work

o prefer a contained workspace

o want a warning (e.g. e-mail) before having face-to-face meetings.

You are a Bystander at work if you:

o are easy-going and not offended by things that others may react to

o miss meetings or deadlines sometimes

o work better with project partners and reminders.

You are a Sensor at work if you:

o want precise directions about work

o prefer structured work projects with details attended to

o want your own work materials.

Strategies for managing work successfully

The three most important issues at work are workspace, work flow, and work relationships. By breaking work into these subsections, it is easier to see how to manage sensory patterns at work.

Managing workspaces with senses in mind

The settings for work are large contributors to our ability to be productive and satisfied there. As you have learned in previous chapters, there will not be one type of workspace that will be satisfying for everyone. We need to select and design workspaces to meet everyone's individual sensory needs.

For Seekers, workspaces can be flexible because changes in the space will keep the Seeker interested. Seekers may keep their work activities out rather than store things, because this will enable the Seeker to encounter their projects and be reminded of what needs to be done. Seekers may also move their furniture about to keep things interesting, so sharing spaces has to be worked out. Seekers will do better with other Seekers or Bystanders in their workspace. Peggy and Don in the story above used workspaces very actively. Let's consider another example of a Seeker at work.

Francine is a buyer for a large department store. She has an assigned workspace, but she is rarely there. She spends a lot of time on the sales floor watching what products are attracting customers and talking to sales staff. She also spends a lot of time on the computer and phone, and traveling to shows to see what is new. She likes to work at the local coffee shop sometimes and in the diner down the street so she can see her friends and neighbors throughout the day.

Bystanders will be casual about their workspaces. Things may remain out on counters, desks, and other surfaces, and may become part of the "background" workspace (i.e. won't be reminders of projects). They won't notice changes in the office easily, and will become aware of them much later than others in the department. Bystanders will be more productive if their workspaces are in the midst of activity; the interruptions will keep the Bystander alert and productive. Inconvenient entrances and exits are also good space management strategies for Bystanders.

Fred caused Tracy to win the office pool. When Fred was out of town, the new conference room chairs arrived and were installed. Charles made a grid with all the meeting dates for the next month, and everyone picked a day when they thought Fred would notice the chairs. Tracy guessed right: it took three weeks and nine meetings for Fred to notice the chairs; everyone was giving him hints when it was their day, but everyone had agreed not to mention the chairs directly. Fred laughed with everyone else because he knew how wild it was that he had sat in the chairs without noticing their new feel.

Sensors will want to have some control over their immediate workspaces, and will want to place themselves so that others have a hard time interfering with the Sensor's workspace. Sensors will have an organizational structure for their supplies, and will tidy up their spaces regularly. Although Sensors will want to have access to others during the work day, they will move into and out of shared spaces to get their own work accomplished.

Katrina works in a busy office. Although everyone has their own offices (a few part-timers share offices), people work with their doors open most of the time. Katrina loves to know what is going on, but is continuously struggling with the noise from the hall as everyone moves about and chats with each other at doorways. She has to close her door for portions of each day to get anything accomplished.

It is the Avoiders who will want isolated workspaces. They will close their door in an office, work at home when possible, or find remote locations for completing activities. Avoiders will have a strong internal plan for their workspace, but it might not be completely evident to an onlooker. Materials might be out, but exposed materials will be part of an overall plan for using the space to complete the work. Avoiders will be intolerant of changes to their workspaces, and productivity will suffer until the Avoider's particular space plan is restored.

Everett is a customer service representative at a neighborhood bank, so he has a desk right on the bank lobby floor. People move in and out of the bank all day, and when they need personalized assistance, they sit at his desk. They have to speak quietly and the manager expects Everett to keep his desk clear so only that person's accounts are on the desk. Everett can't imagine working any other way; this is a quiet, tidy, organized job, and his desk keeps a good space between him and his customers.

Sometimes co-workers have to spend time together in a confined space.

Louisa and Ruth were assigned to a project that required a monthly road trip. It was only logical for them to drive together, but logic wasn't all they needed to make it through these trips. Louisa loved being on the road, and would crank up the radio and sing (badly) when she had long drives. Ruth liked to use the drives as a peaceful meditative time. At first, they didn't talk about this, and whoever was driving did what they wanted with the radio, but then as they got further into the project, this contrast started to grate on their collective nerves:

"That radio is getting on my last nerve; I need to think about our meeting when we get there, and I cannot concentrate with you and the radio blaring." (Ruth)

"The music helps me release my inhibitions so I can be more creative when we get to the meeting!" (Louisa)

What a dilemma for these co-workers! The very things they each need are clashing together. Luckily, they had high regard for each other on the project, and negotiated a plan. Louisa brought her ipod along on the road trips, and agreed to practice humming and singing softly so Ruth could drown out her singing with some jazz on the radio. They also agreed that they would use part of each trip to prepare for the meeting, so they wouldn't have as much time in these different music/thinking zones. On the way home, they would debrief about the meeting before retreating into their music zones.

Managing work flow and schedules with senses in mind

All types of work require attention to time in some manner. Construction work has schedules for each phase; plumbers and electricians need to negotiate with carpenters about whose turn it is to work on a space. Work in schools ebb and flow with semesters, finals, and graduation. Offices have peak and average times for deadlines that must be met. How we manage the work flow in any of these situations is dependent on our sensory patterns.

Seekers and Bystanders will be flexible with their schedules

Seekers and Bystanders will be flexible with their schedules, and it will not be apparent to others how they are meeting their time deadlines. Seekers and Bystanders can handle emergencies more easily because of their flexibility. Even though a seeker may have scheduled a time to work on a project, if something else catches the Seeker's interest, the scheduled activity will be abandoned to work on the new ideas. For Bystanders, time will be more likely to drift away, with the Bystander suddenly noticing that it is time to get to a meeting (or that they missed one). Seekers and Bystanders can either work at the last minute on projects that are due, or can even be late because of their "flexible" attitude about time.

Table 7: Examples of harnessing
sensory patterns for work productivity

Sensory behavior	Which can be challenging because...	We can harness the behavior positively...
Seeker behavior		
Spontaneous and creative	It disrupts the schedule for work	Assign Seekers to new product development teams
	It creates a chaotic work environment	Include Seekers on trouble-shooting projects
Work on multiple projects at the same time	It interferes with others being able to move a project forward in a timely manner	Involve Seekers in idea generation and develop-ment and hand projects over to others for imple-mentation
	It creates a cluttered workspace	Provide a separate "cre-ative" space
Bystander behavior		
Casual	It creates appearance that work is not important	Assign Bystanders to crisis teams to provide calming influence
	It develops tension about meeting deadlines	Create physical schedules for the Bystander to refer-ence
Misses meetings	Work doesn't get completed	Create an alarm system to remind Bystander of meetings
	It "wastes" others' time	Get another team member to stop by and get the Bystander for the meetings

Sensory behavior	Which can be challenging because...	We can harness the behavior positively...
Avoider behavior		
Very structured work plans and timelines	People have different ideas about how the work needs to be done	Assign Avoider to complete infrastructure work in a project
	When something goes wrong, rigidity can interfere with problem solving	Place Avoider in charge of planning training on procedures, particularly related to safety
Isolated work patterns	It makes for difficult meetings and negotiations	Create e-mail groups for projects so Avoider can "communicate" without having face-to-face contact
	It slows down work process trying to get answers back	Assign the Avoider the parts of the project that require the least human contact
Sensor behavior		
Prefers to have own materials and supplies	It creates territoriality It harbors mistrust	Provide supplies/materials work stations or bins so everyone can access their "own" materials
		Color-code materials/ supplies so an entire set of materials stay together
Precise and detail-oriented	Pickiness can wear people down	Assign Sensor to final edits on behalf of whole team
	It creates a sense of feeling that nothing is good enough	Reorganize work so checking details is the Sensor's assigned work for others, and let the Sensor fix the materials, not just notice the needed changes

Sensors and Avoiders will be
structured with their schedules
. . . .

Sensors and Avoiders will be structured with their schedules, planning carefully for deadlines. They are an asset to time-driven work productivity and can be valuable members of teams if they have the responsibility for scheduled products. However, the schedule can become a tyrant for Sensors and Avoiders, such that when other emergencies come along, they have a difficult time handling the interruption to their schedule. Productivity can suffer from both the emergency not being handled and from the disruption getting them out of the flow of the work they expected to do.

Managing work relationships with senses in mind

In Chapter 5, we discussed work relationships as well as personal relationships. Whenever more than one human being has a common interest or goal, negotiations must take place to meet everyone's needs. Meeting sensory needs is no exception.

It is very easy to become irritated with people at work who have different sensory patterns from our own. Seekers tend to be flamboyant (which they find quite charming about themselves), which can be quite bothersome behavior for Sensors who are trying to manage the amount of sensory input they have to contend with. Avoiders who create structure can be viewed as stifling the creativity of Seekers who want to brainstorm and free associate. Bystanders might seem uninterested in a project to a Sensor who has it all precisely planned out.

So how do we harness each person's natural sensory pattern tendencies to increase work satisfaction and productivity? Table 7 provides some examples to get your thinking started.

The stock department at the grocery store needs many workers to keep the store full for the customers. When working with the stock manager, we looked at sensory patterns that might be a good match for the different tasks. After a discussion, we agreed that an employee who is a Seeker might be a good person to float, that is, to move through the store to pick up items that have been left in the wrong places and return them to their proper shelves. Sensor employees might be great at shelf placement, making sure that everything is precisely lined up on the shelves. Avoiders might work best in the back room unpacking the deliveries, partnered with Bystanders who can cross-check the packing lists to make sure everything arrived.

Special considerations for work

We acknowledge that we each have strengths because of our sensory patterns, and also have challenges because of our sensory patterns. Here are some tips to take advantage of your strengths and minimize the effects of your challenges in sensory processing at work:

Tips for Seekers

- Ask to be assigned to projects requiring creative thinking.

- Offer to brainstorm solutions when problems arise.

- Ask people if they want some ideas before offering them.

- Negotiate changes in your assigned work when new opportunities come up (instead of letting things slide because you get caught up in a new project).

- Look for Sensors and Avoiders on your work teams to help you organize your projects.

- Create a color coding or bin system for keeping projects out and still organized.

Tips for Bystanders

- Find external strategies for reminding you of meeting times and deadlines.

- Identify a buddy on your work team to remind you of things.

- Use the alarm on your computer or PDA.

- Keep work out (and in colorful containers) so you encounter things you are supposed to be working on.

- Wear an ipod while working to keep stimulated.

- Look for Sensors and Avoiders to help you organize projects.

- Look for Seekers to keep you stimulated during work.

- Find different ways to get to places at work.

- Accept assignments on highly charged work teams because you will provide calm and be stimulated at the same time.

Tips for Avoiders

- Select work and projects that require a high degree of structure and organization.

- Identify the one-person tasks on projects, and volunteer for those tasks.

- Offer to work in the remote locations that others may not want.

- Work at home when you can.

- Use e-mail to reduce the number of people stopping by your work area.

- Let Seekers come up with ideas to enhance your projects and you take over when the implementation is required.

- Serve on safety and procedure committees.

- Schedule one or two blocks of time for people to meet with you so they are not bugging you all the time.

Tips for Sensors

- Identify a designated workspace for yourself even if it is very small, and focus on this being the area you have control over.

- Put up a sign that indicates when you are available for drop-in or scheduled appointments.

- Volunteer to do final checks/edits of work for your work team.

- Be very careful about how much you schedule each day.

- "Schedule" some flexible time each day for unexpected things.

- Offer to be the scribe/note person at a meeting to be sure everything gets recorded properly.

- Design some safety valve strategies for getting away when things get overwhelming (errands, getting a drink, taking a walk).

11

Sensational Leisure and Recreation: Let's Get Personal

Leisure time is personal time; time to unwind and recharge. That is where the similarity about leisure from person to person ends. Every person has a different idea about what is relaxing. Your sensory patterns contribute to what makes something relaxing or not. In our opening story, the Zimmer family learns that the *idea* of a vacation, *planning* a vacation, and the *implementation* of the vacation can be very different matters; not all of them are relaxing.

Opening story

Road trip?!

It is very early in the morning, and actually still looks like night-time outside. Priscilla Zimmer is waking her family so they can get a good start on their day. This is the beginning of their vacation; they are driving for two days to a neighboring state that has many sights they want to see.

Her husband, Gideon, doesn't awaken easily, so she has turned on the lights and TV, and moved on to get the kids up. Her daughter, Hilda, is already awake and sitting on the side of her bed. Priscilla smiles to herself; she thinks that Hilda must be excited about their trip. Rudy is still asleep, but awakens pretty quickly when she comes into his room.

As they are pulling out of the driveway, Gideon realizes that he didn't put his duffle in the car, so they go back to get it. And then they are off! Priscilla has the maps marked with the route, has snacks for everyone (their favorites, this is their *vacation*!), and is ready to be the perfect navigator.

As the sun is rising, so are the tempers in the car. In the back seat, Hilda is upset by Rudy's continuous activity. He has earphones on his CD player, but is playing it so loudly that she can hear every note. He is humming, drumming, and dancing to every song. He also has coloring books, puzzle books, and a game machine on the seat, and they keep sliding into her. She uses her pillows to create a fortress, but they are no match for Rudy's things.

There are challenges in the front seat too. Gideon has missed two turns despite Priscilla's advance directions. Gideon tried to make these wrong turns into adventures, pointing out what they have been able to see because of the detours. Priscilla remains focused on the time delay they have because of the errors and is agitated by the traffic they now have to contend with. The tension from the children in the back seat isn't helping Priscilla's mood either and what makes things worse for her is that Gideon seems oblivious to what is going on.

Believe it or not, the Zimmers had a lot of fun planning what they would be doing on their vacation, and enjoyed reading about places and picking their favorites. The process of finding out information was easier for them than this early part of their trip. During planning, they had more flexibility about how, where, and when they would find out about their options. Hilda went to the library because she could hole up in a quiet corner to read about the attractions. Rudy used the Internet while text messaging with his friends, and found some instant chats that would answer his questions about the attractions. Priscilla perused books and pamphlets while her family was getting ready in the morning; she got distracted when Rudy arrived in the kitchen so it took her two weeks to get through everything. Gideon just listened to everyone's comments during and after dinner time each night.

Does this situation sound familiar? When family members have leisure time together, fun can be harder to come by than we think. If we look at this situation from a sensory processing point of view, the situation makes a little more sense. During the planning phase, each family member could construct their situations themselves, thus being able to meet their own personal needs while imagining their vacation. However, when they started the trip, they were restrained in the car together.

Priscilla is a Sensor; we can see that she gets overwhelmed quickly (like getting distracted in the kitchen, in the car with the traffic and her children). She tries to manage situations so she doesn't get overwhelmed (having the maps and snacks ready), but this doesn't help sometimes. Hilda also gets overwhelmed easily, but as an Avoider, she retreats. She found an isolated place to do her research, but cannot get away from her brother in the car. Rudy, a Seeker, is full of activity, which is a really bad match for Hilda in the back seat of the car. Gideon is a Bystander and so seems easy-going and sometimes oblivious depending on your perspective. He doesn't detect all the sensory experiences that are going on around him. This is good in that he isn't ruffled when driving, but this also leads to him missing the signs for turns he needs to make.

So, it might be a better strategy for Rudy to sit in the front seat with Gideon. Rudy's antics would not only *not* be bothersome to his dad, they might also keep Gideon more alert while driving. If Gideon and Rudy interact, this might be helpful too. This would leave the back seat to Hilda and Priscilla who might create a little haven for themselves. They would be less physically active, and would be likely to keep their own spaces distinct and comfortable. Rudy might be assigned the task of looking for the signs for the turns, giving dad more cues about directions. These simple changes could create a better beginning to this long-anticipated leisure time for the Zimmers as a family unit.

Introduction

Sensory patterns affect our leisure choices as much as they affect other parts of our lives. People think about leisure time with fondness. People spend a lot of time planning what they want to do, how to spend time relaxing, and where leisure ought to take place.

Many factors contribute to our leisure choices. We each have special interests, skills, and talents that shape our ideas about what leisure will be for ourselves. Sensory patterns will also affect our choices. Avoiders will gravitate toward quiet singular activities, while Seekers will opt for intensely social or physical activities. Sensors will want to plan precise leisure time, and will have a few chosen activities, while Bystanders may meander their way into leisure time.

The most important principle to remember is that leisure is *your* time to unwind, change pace, and feel satisfied and refreshed. Following this principle means that you have to pick activities that are a great match for your sensory patterns; by meeting your sensory needs, you contribute to an overall sense of satisfaction. Leisure needs to recharge you, and your sensory systems can be a great vehicle for revitalization.

We have a substantial body of data and case studies demonstrating that our personal interests might guide us towards activities that may or may not meet our sensory needs. By understanding sensory patterns, we can shape the way we engage in leisure. Let's discuss some of the major categories of leisure and how we can tailor them to meet individual needs of people in every sensory pattern.

Vacationing

The opening story describes a family vacation. Many people have had vacations that were very different during the planning than during the actual vacation. At home, people construct ways to get what they need (e.g. retreating to a bedroom, going out with friends, turning on music), but vacations have unfamiliar surroundings, schedules, and activities. Without a clear idea about how to meet sensory needs, these unfamiliar settings can be difficult.

Planning with family or friends regarding the vacation and discussing what would make the time the most enjoyable can provide helpful information. Daily life routines provide a clue about how people get their sensory needs met every day; incorporating these strategies into vacationing makes it possible to meet needs in new places. For some families, taking some vacation time separately works because the time is tailored to meet people's exact needs; remember that vacations are for rejuvenating.

Seekers might select a new place to explore; Bystanders will be open to lots of options and may just take off for an unknown location. Avoiders might pick a cabin in one location, and Sensors are likely to plan a specific schedule for their activities.

Travel

In the story of the Zimmers, they traveled in their car. People also travel by plane to many locations. Planes are very contained places with lots of people in them, so sensory needs getting met is a challenge. The cramped space of an airplane is a likely spot for clashing of sensations. People are pushed to the edge of their capacity for politeness in this situation, and this always brings out everyone's needs. With attention and vigilance, it is possible.

Meg is returning from a foreign country, so the trip is going to be long and cramped for everyone. Since Meg is a Seeker, she brings lots of things to keep her system fed with sensory input for the eight-hour flight. She has two books, some cross-stitching, folders from her office, a crossword puzzle book, a CD/DVD player, and some photos she wants to organize. Meg is thrilled she got an aisle seat (which means she can see what is going on up and down the aisle), *and* the middle seat is vacant, creating more space for her activities. She wonders whether she will be able to talk to the person in the window seat.

Her row companion is Jaime. Jaime is an Avoider; he requested a window seat so that he would not have to be bumped repeatedly as people go up and down the aisle during the flight. He waited until the end of boarding so he could get on the plane without the crowd around him. As Jaime approaches his row, a man is standing in the aisle arranging his belongings in his seat area across from Meg. Although many other people were also in the aisle, which meant that they wouldn't be taking off any time soon, Jaime becomes more uncomfortable as time passes, and insists that the man stop his activities so he could get out of the aisle and into his seat.

Once Jaime is seated, he proceeds to build himself a fortress for the trip. He puts his book about the country they are going to in his seat pocket, and props up his watch (which has two faces for two time zones on it), slides his perfectly sized bag under the seat, stows a water bottle next to his bag, puts earplugs into his ears, removes his shoes, lines them up carefully, and puts on a new pair of socks. Meg watches in amazement (of course she is watching, she is a Seeker!), and thinks to herself "This man should be the star in a 'how to get seated for your flight' video."

Jaime continues to sit perfectly square in his seat; Meg rotates her legs so they move into the unused middle seat space. Jaime takes out one thing at a time throughout the flight, while Meg sprawls several of her items onto the empty seat, and shifts from one to another throughout the flight.

If you identify with Jaime, you are saying "This man has his act together!" Avoiders can be challenged by the contained space of an airplane because they will have to encounter sounds from other people and the plane, touch from the closeness of other people, smells from food and drinks, continuous movement of other passengers, and they cannot get away from all this. Avoiders value routines and order because the sensations are familiar in routine situations. Avoiders can reduce the amount of sensation by planning as much as possible. In the plane story, Jaime is creating a planned space away from areas that might disrupt his order.

If you identify with Meg, you are saying "This woman has her act together!" Seekers can be very challenged by the contained space of an airplane because they need a variety of activities to keep themselves satisfied, and on long flights, the plane can be restraining to the Seeker's need to move around, explore new things, and experiment with new opportunities. Seekers value variety, and so have to bring some of the variety with them to have a successful flight (especially a long flight). In the plane story, Meg is providing herself with many opportunities so she can change around during the flight.

This could be a volatile situation. Although Meg and Jaime are both working to get their sensory needs met during the flight, they could clash as they try to manage in their own ways. Although their strategies are in sharp contrast to each other, they share the same objective of getting their sensory needs met so they can have the best flight possible. When we understand the reasons why people might be handling a challenging situation differently from ourselves, we have a better chance to help each other through the harder spots. If Meg sees that Jaime may be overwhelmed by the sensory experiences of the plane, then she might not talk to him as much, or manage her activities more carefully. Jaime, seeing the differences between himself and Meg, could let her know that it is OK to put some of her things on the extra seat, explaining that he is just glad not to have another person there. When we can identify the sensory needs that others are trying to meet, we can be good stewards of each other.

Free time at home

What do people choose to do with their free time at home? Typically people select activities that make them feel the most satisfied or fulfilled. Free time in the midst of a busy life needs to be rejuvenating, so free time choices provide a window into how sensory needs are met. When people get depleted during free time, it is possible that the activities are not consistent with the person's sensory needs.

Linda drives her husband crazy at home. When they say they are going to have a leisurely evening at home watching a movie, Orlando envisions getting into his comfortable sweatpants and snuggling into the couch for the evening. He likes to turn out the lights so it is more like the theatre, and all the attention can be on the TV screen. He has learned that this is a fantasy for him, because it doesn't work out this way with Linda. She loves to watch movies with Orlando too, but she gets too antsy just sitting there staring at the screen. She gets out her stitching so she can sew while watching the movie. Of course, this means she has to have her magnifying light on so she can see the detail work; the light makes a glare on the screen, so Orlando has rearranged the furniture to stop that distraction. Linda looks at the screen in between stitches, so sometimes misses an important part of the story, and so she is regularly asking Orlando what just happened. Linda also gets up a lot during the movie, to go to the bathroom, to get a drink, to make a snack. Orlando does not see the "relaxing" part of this type of evening for Linda, and Linda cannot imagine how Orlando can just sit there for two hours without crawling out of his skin.

Obviously, Linda is a Seeker; this means that she needs to add other things to the experience of "watching a movie" in order to feel relaxed. This might not make sense to others who are not Seekers (Orlando, for instance), but for Linda, moving around and doing something with her hands while watching the movie create just the right amount of sensory input to keep Linda settled. Orlando's strategies of reducing additional sensory input to really focus on the movie (good strategies for Avoiders) also reduce input to an unacceptable level for Linda. Rearranging the seating was a good idea to keep Linda's movements from distracting Orlando.

Physical activities

There is a wide range of physical activities that can meet the needs of people in all sensory patterns. There are several factors to consider before making a decision about how satisfying a physical activity will be for each person. First, consider the amount and type of sensory input available through the physical activity. Next, consider the conditions or environments in which a person might engage in the physical activity, because environments change the available sensory input.

Think about running. Running provides a lot of sensory input to the feet, joints, and muscles of the legs. This intense sensory input might be attractive to a Seeker; however, the rhythmic, predictable, and repetitive nature of running might also be attractive to an Avoider. A Seeker might choose running in a busy gym or a densely populated neighborhood, and an Avoider might choose running in a home gym or on a quiet street. Bystanders might do better when running on paths that vary (thus keeping their attention focused on the changes occurring around them), while Sensors may prefer the predictability of running on a treadmill that provides even and steady input.

There are certainly physical activities that are more likely choices for Seekers, Avoiders, and so on. Seekers are more likely to choose rock climbing, Avoiders are more likely to choose meditating, Sensors are more likely to choose an organized exercise class, and Bystanders are more likely to choose activities that fit into their daily routines (like walking a longer way to the car rather than planning something as "exercise").

But even each of these activities could be placed in a setting that would make them attractive to a person with another sensory pattern. Perhaps rock climbing creates for an Avoider a place of solitude (no one else can get around you when you get to that ledge!). With a challenging yoga position, meditation might be very attractive to a Seeker. A Sensor might have a set place to park the car so there is a predetermined walk built into the day. And a Bystander might join a friend in a class. So it is the personal construction of physical activities and leisure time that makes them both satisfying to the sensory systems and to meeting leisure interests.

Ling loves to ski and plans a trip every winter. She has become pretty skilled at skiing, so it is common for her to ski the more difficult slopes. She had a weird experience last winter:

> We have this certain lodge that we like to go to, so we were skiing familiar slopes. As we ascended on the lift, it was like we went through the clouds when flying on an airplane. The air was like pea soup, only white! I started skiing down the mountain, and I fell several times in the first couple of minutes. It was like I had never skied before. I couldn't figure out where I was going, and couldn't get my body, arms, and legs to get into auto-pilot and *ski*. After I got below that cloud

cover, I was fine. I realized that I need to *see* what I am doing; my eyes must be in charge of my skiing; how funny!

Skiing might generally be more desirable for people who seek movement. What Ling learned in her ski experience is that her visual system is her strong guidance system for skiing, and that her body position system relies on visual guidance and monitoring to function (even though she wouldn't explain it this way!). Perhaps the fast moving visual world as she skis down the mountain is what she is seeking. Other skiers use the body position system to direct their skiing, with visual input a support to this primary function. With this second kind of skier, we would hear more about how the joints feel as they adjust during skiing. This person might be seeking body position input, with skiing as a great way to get that input.

Entertainment

Events can provide leisure as well. Everyone has ideas about optimal entertainment options; these options have sensory characteristics that can make them attractive to people with different sensory patterns. Small, quiet venues will attract Avoiders and Sensors, while large, crowded venues will attract Seekers and Bystanders. Seekers and Bystanders will be more open to attending events with unknown performers or experimental topics, while Avoiders and Sensors will choose their favorites. Planning will be more attractive to Sensors, while spontaneity will increase satisfaction for Seekers.

Entertainment can also be at home. Music, TV, and computer games create entertainment options as well. As with other forms of entertainment, it is not who will listen to music, watch TV, or play on the computer, but how each of us might approach these activities. There is music for everyone: quiet, predictable rhythms for Avoiders, edgy sounds for Seekers, formula music for Sensors, and mixes for Bystanders.

Think of your choices and the choices of friends and family from a sensory point of view; how is each of you meeting your needs? When you need to negotiate entertainment with a friend or family member, think about how you can find common ground. For example, perhaps you agree to watch a sporting event at home rather than at a crowded bar to accommodate Sensors and Avoiders in your group, but have food in the kitchen to enable Seekers and Bystanders to move around during the game.

Resting

Yes, resting is a leisure activity! You are reading this thinking, "What is there to talk about? We all know what resting is." But think a little longer. Some people need quiet to be able to nap. If your child wants to watch TV in the next room, how soft does the TV have to be before you will be able to get to sleep? Or do you need to go to another part of the house to be able to nap?

When you get home from work and need to rest for 30 minutes before dinner, what does resting mean for you? Do you want to sit and be quiet, do some knitting, go for a run, make a snack in the kitchen, read the paper? Each of these choices reflects some sensory needs being met. Sitting quietly might be very satisfying for a Sensor, but a Seeker might get more agitated just sitting, and would add knitting to the sitting to feel calmer (because getting more sensory input makes a Seeker feel more satisfied).

Bianca's idea of the perfect day off is to go to the most remote area of the park with a blanket, a book, a thermos of tea, and her music. She carefully sets up her space to make sure nothing pokes through the blanket to bug her, and then she nestles in to go on whatever adventure the book has in store for her. She is so mellow at the end of her day, she feels like she has been on a vacation but without the hassle of traveling.

Bianca is a Sensor; she understands that creating just the right amount of input can be satisfying for her. Reading in a quiet place with the gentle smells of nature and soothing music are perfect for her. She also knows that she needs to be careful about things touching her skin, so she plans for that as well.

Hanging out

A related relaxation activity is hanging out. People might hang out in a coffee shop, at a restaurant or bar, on the deck or in the yard, or in a more exotic location (like on a beach, or a mountain). There are many options for hanging out in each of these venues. Many types of coffee shops exist; some are quiet and out of the way, while others are a buzz of activity. People can enter and exit quickly or they can linger in the environment. So it is not the venue per se that makes it satisfying for a particular person, but the way a person uses the venue that reveals how they are going to get their sensory needs met.

Rose and Morgan have made an art out of hanging out. They are both 20-somethings who live in the heart of their city. They really like hanging out in very crowded bars, dance halls, or coffee houses where they will see many people during the evening. These are command performance events for them, and they spend a lot of time picking out just the right look from their wardrobes. So we would guess that Rose and Morgan are Seekers with the high-intensity environments they are selecting. These venues would be completely overwhelming to a Sensor or Avoider, who would want to choose quiet, cozy venues.

Sometimes, however, they also want to go to the quiet, dark corner of the neighborhood coffee shop so they can "chill" and catch up on their lives. For these times, they love wearing their low-maintenance clothing: sweats, flip flops, and a pony tail. So then, these women switch on us, and go to the very places that we would expect Sensors and Avoiders to choose, and Seekers to stay away from. This is the interesting twist to leisure—people make settings work for them. In the quiet neighborhood coffee shop, Morgan and Rose are talking a mile a minute, interrupting each other as they go, weaving through the conversation throughout their time together. They are probably also changing their seating position repeatedly during the visit. A Sensor or Avoider would use the coffee shop as a quiet respite to get away from other people, sit in one place and read, or daydream. They would *not* like sitting near Morgan and Rose if they are going into the coffee house to regroup. So it is the personal touch we add to our hanging out that makes it restful for each of us.

Reading and puzzles

On first consideration, reading might seem like a more passive type of recreation, and therefore more attractive to Sensors and Avoiders. These individuals will want to find a special place for reading, and the topics they choose to read may reflect a more calming influence. Seekers may change where they read frequently, read in bursts, and read books that provide vicarious sensory pleasures. Seekers and Bystanders might peruse magazines for new ideas, and look through magazines several times, noticing different things each time. Sensors and Avoiders will go through the magazine systematically, reading it in order from front to back. Newspaper reading might be similar, with Bystanders and Seekers taking a more random approach (pulling out favorite sections, "messing up the paper for others"), while Sensors and Avoiders would want to progress systematically through the paper "the right way."

Puzzles (e.g. crossword, sudoku, solitaire) can also be satisfying for people in every sensory pattern depending on how they are used. Sensors and Avoiders may be more systematic, while Seekers and Bystanders may approach these tasks more randomly (e.g. jumping around, starting and stopping, making cross outs all over the page). The same issue of settings applies: quiet isolated places versus busy environments.

Creative projects

Creative endeavors are very sacred to people. We choose art and craft projects, gardening, decorating, and cooking as means of expressing ourselves. Because creative endeavors reflect who we are, they are also great things to get our sensory needs met. Interests and sensory needs intersect to support our creative projects. Many people choose cooking as a leisure activity interest, but the way people cook will reflect sensory patterns. Sensors will follow the directions more precisely, while Seekers will estimate and experiment with the recipes. Bystanders will also be more easy-going about the recipes, and may forget some ingredients, and will continue to enjoy the experience. Avoiders who like cooking will perfect specific recipes that are their favorites.

Summary

Leisure is very personal, so building sensory patterns into decision-making increases the chances that leisure will be satisfying and pleasurable. Leisure must be rejuvenating, so it must also be consistent with sensory needs. If a leisure activity leaves you feeling depleted, then perhaps it reflects an interest area, but is not respectful of your sensory needs.

Willie loves numbers, so is excited to hear about sudoku puzzles. A colleague at work introduces him to the game by giving him a starter book. Willie tries one on a break at work as he sits in the break room. He gets interrupted several times, and finds the whole experience frustrating.

At home that night, he decides to try again. He works on another puzzle from the book as he eats his dinner, and gets totally into the flow of the puzzle. Four puzzles later, he pulls himself away to get the dishes cleaned up.

Willie is an Avoider for sounds, so the break room depletes him even with a favored activity. When he changes venues, he can enjoy the activity.

Leisure and recreation checklist

- o Your leisure activity reflects a personal interest.

- o You feel re-energized after the activity.

- o The place you select makes it more satisfying.

- o Your recreation activity happens on your terms.

- o Your leisure and recreation time are consistent with your sensory needs.

Final thoughts

In this book, you have learned how to crack the sensory code for yourself and your family and friends. You have also learned how special circumstances can bring out different reactions because of their characteristics. You now have many ideas about how to adjust living situations to meet everyone's sensory needs, and create a more harmonious living, working, and leisure space.

Remember, each person is completely unique, and therefore has certain distinct ways of responding in life. We could not cover every possible pattern in this book; I hope I provided you with enough examples and ideas to enable you to crack individual sensory codes that you encounter in yourself and those around you. The more you practice, the better you will get, and the more harmonious life will be for everyone!

Get cracking!
Enjoy your sensational life!

Bibliography

Studies validating sensory patterns (using the Sensory Profile measures)

Brown, C. and Dunn, W. (2002) *The Adolescent/Adult Sensory Profile Manual.* San Antonio, TX: Psychological Corporation.

Brown, T., Cromwell, R., Filion, D., Dunn, W. and Tollefson, N. (2002) 'Sensory Processing in Schizophrenia: Missing and Avoiding Information.' *Schizophrenia Research 55*, 1–2, 187–195.

Brown, C., Tollefson, N., Dunn, W., Cromwell, R. and Filion, D. (2001) 'The Adult Sensory Profile: Measuring Patterns of sensory processing.' *American Journal of Occupational Therapy 55*, 1, 75–82.

Dove, S. (2003) 'Sensory Processing in Children Who Have Specific Learning Disabilities.' *Masters Thesis: University of Kansas.*

Dunn, W. (1997) 'The Impact of Sensory Processing Abilities on the Daily Lives of Young Children and Families: A Conceptual Model.' *Infants and Young Children 9*, 4, 23–35.

Dunn, W. (1999) *The Sensory Profile Manual.* San Antonio, TX: Psychological Corporation.

Dunn, W. (2002) *The Infant/Toddler Sensory Profile.* San Antonio, TX: Psychological Corporation.

Dunn, W. (2006a) *Sensory Profile School Companion.* San Antonio, TX: Psychological Corporation.

Dunn, W. (2006b) *Sensory Profile Supplement.* San Antonio, TX: Psychological Corporation.

Dunn, W. and Bennett, D. (2002) 'Patterns of Sensory Processing in Children with Attention Deficit Hyperactivity Disorder.' *Occupational Therapy Journal of Research 22*, 1, 4–15.

Dunn, W. and Brown, C. (1997) 'Factor Analysis on the Sensory Profile from a National Sample of Children without Disabilities.' *American Journal of Occupational Therapy 51*, 7, 490–495.

Dunn, W. and Daniels, D. (2001) 'Initial Development of the Infant/Toddler Sensory Profile.' *Journal of Early Intervention 25*, 1, 27–41.

Dunn, W. and Westman, K. (1997) 'The Sensory Profile: The Performance of a National Sample of Children Without Disabilities.' *American Journal of Occupational Therapy 51*, 1, 25–34.

Dunn, W., Myles, B. and Orr, S. (2002) 'Sensory Processing Issues Associated with Asperger Syndrome: A Preliminary Investigation.' *American Journal of Occupational Therapy 56*, 1, 97–102.

Dunn, W., Saiter, J. and Rinner, L. (2002) 'Asperger Syndrome and Sensory Processing: A Conceptual Model and Guidance for Intervention Planning.' *Focus on Autism and other Developmental Disabilities 17*, 3, 172–185.

Ermer, J. and Dunn, W. (1998) 'The Sensory Profile: A Discriminant Analysis of Children With and Without Disabilities.' *American Journal of Occupational Therapy 52*, 4, 283–290.

Kientz, M.A. and Dunn, W. (1997) 'Comparison of the Performance of Children with and Without Autism on the Sensory Profile.' *American Journal of Occupational Therapy 51*, 7, 530–537.

McIntosh, D.N., Miller, L.J., Shyu, V. and Dunn, W. (1999) 'Overview of the Short Sensory Profile (SSP).' In W. Dunn (ed.) *The Sensory Profile Manual.* San Antonio, TX: Psychological Corporation, pp.59–74.

Myles, B.S., Hagiwara, T., Dunn, W., Rinner, L., Reese, M., Huggins, A. *et al.* (2004) 'Sensory Issues in Children with Asperger Syndrome and Autism.' *Education and Training in Developmental Disabilities 3*, 4, 283–290.

Pohl, P., Dunn, W. and Brown, C. (2001) 'The Role of Sensory Processing in the Everyday Lives of Older Adults.' *Occupational Therapy Journal of Research 23*, 3, 99–106.

Rogers, S., Hepburn, S. and Wehner, E. (2003) 'Parent Report of Sensory Symptoms in Toddlers with Autism and Those with Other Developmental Disorders.' *Journal of Autism and Developmental Disorders 33*, 6, 631–642.

Watling, R., Dietz, J. and White, O. (2001) 'Comparison of Sensory Profile Scores of Young Children With and Without Autism Spectrum Disorders.' *American Journal of Occupational Therapy 55*, 4, 416–423.

Background reading

Aron, E.N. and Aron, A. (1997) 'Sensory-processing Sensitivity and Its Relation to Introversion and Emotionality.' *Journal of Personality and Social Psychology 73*, 2, 345–368.

Ayres, A.J. (1979) *Sensory Integration and the Child.* Los Angeles: Western Psychological Services.

Ayres, A.J. (1989) *Sensory Integration and Praxis Tests.* Los Angeles: Western Psychological Services.

Ayres, A.J. and Tickle, L.S. (1980) 'Hyper-responsivity to Touch and Vestibular Stimuli as Predictor of Positive Response to Sensory Integration Procedures by Autistic Children.' *American Journal of Occupational Therapy 34*, 6, 375–381.

Baranek, G.T. (1999) 'Autism During Infancy: A Retrospective Video Analysis of Sensory-motor and Social Behaviors at 9–12 Months of Age.' *Journal of Autism and Developmental Disorders 29*, 3, 213–224.

Baranek, G.T. (2002) 'Efficacy of Sensory and Motor Interventions for Children with Autism.' *Journal of Autism and Developmental Disorders 32*, 5, 397–422.

Baranek, G.T., Foster, L.G. and Berkson, G. (1997) 'Sensory Defensiveness in Persons with Developmental Disabilities.' *Occupational Therapy Journal of Research 17*, 3, 173–185.

Blanche, E. and Schaaf, R. (2001) 'Proprioception: The Sixth Sense.' In S. Roley, E. Blanche and R. Schaaf (eds) *Sensory Integration with Developmental Disabilities.* San Antonio, TX: Psychological Corporation.

Case-Smith, J. and Bryan, T. (1999) 'The Effects of Occupational Therapy with Sensory Integration Emphasis on Preschool-age Children with Autism.' *American Journal of Occupational Therapy 53,* 5, 489–497.

Case-Smith, J., Butcher, L. and Reed, D. (1998) 'Parents' Report of Sensory Responsiveness and Temperament in Preterm Infants.' *American Journal of Occupational Therapy 52,* 7, 547–555.

Cohn, E.S. and Cermak, S.A. (1998) 'Including the Family Perspective in Sensory Integration Outcomes Research.' *American Journal of Occupational Therapy 52,* 7, 540–546.

Cohn, E., Miller, L.J. and Tickle-Degnen, L. (2000) 'Parental Hopes for Therapy Outcomes: Children with Sensory Modulation Disorders.' *American Journal of Occupational Therapy 54,* 1, 36–43.

Cooper, J., Majnemer, A., Rosenblatt, B. and Birnbaum, R. (1993) 'A Standardized Sensory Assessment for Children of School-age.' *Physical and Occupational Therapy in Pediatrics 13,* 1, 61–80.

Coster, W., Tickle-Degnen, L. and Armenta, L. (1995) 'Therapist–Child Interaction During Sensory Integration Treatment: Development and Testing of a Research Tool.' *Occupational Therapy Journal of Research 15,* 1, 17–35.

DeGangi, G.A. and Greenspan, S.I. (1988) 'The Development of Sensory Functions in Infants.' *Physical and Occupational Therapy in Pediatrics 8,* 4, 21–33.

DeGangi, G.A. and Greenspan, S.I. (1989) *Test of Sensory Functions in Infants Manual.* Los Angeles, CA: Western Psychological Services.

Dunbar, S.B. (1999) 'A Child's Occupational Performance: Consideration of Sensory Processing and Family Context.' *American Journal of Occupational Therapy 53,* 2, 231–235.

Dunkerley, E., Tickle-Degnen, L. and Coster, W.J. (1997) 'Therapist–Child Interaction in the Middle Minutes of Sensory Integration Treatment.' *American Journal of Occupational Therapy 51,* 10, 799–805.

Fallon, M.A., Mauer, D.M. and Neukirch, M. (1994) 'The Effectiveness of Sensory Integration Activities on Language Processing in Preschoolers who are Sensory and Language Impaired.' *Infant Toddler Intervention 4,* 3, 235–243.

Fisher, A.G., Murray, E.A. and Bundy, A.C. (1991) *Sensory Integration Theory and Practice.* Philadelphia, PA: F.A. Davis.

Jarus, T. and Gol, D. (1995) 'The Effect of Kinesthetic Stimulation on the Acquisition and Retention of Gross Motor Skill by Children With and Without Sensory Integration Disorders.' *Physical and Occupational Therapy in Pediatrics 14,* 3/4, 59–73.

Jin, Y., Bunney, W.E., Sandman, Jr., C.A., Patterson, J.V., Fleming, K., Moenter, J.R. *et al.* (1998) 'Is P50 Suppression a Measure of Sensory Gating in Schizophrenia?' *Biological Psychiatry 43,* 12, 873–878.

Johnson-Ecker, C.L. and Parham, L.D. (2000) 'The Evaluation of Sensory Processing: A Validity Study Using Contrasting Groups.' *American Journal of Occupational Therapy 54,* 5, 494–503.

Kinnealey, M. (1998) 'Princess or Tyrant: A Case Report of a Child with Sensory Defensiveness.' *Occupational Therapy International 5*, 4, 293–303.

Kinnealey, M. and Fuiek, M. (1999) 'The Relationship Between Sensory Defensiveness, Anxiety, Depression and Perception of Pain in Adults.' *Occupational Therapy International 6*, 3, 195–206.

Kinnealey, M., Oliver, B. and Wilbarger, P. (1995) 'A Phenomenological Study of Sensory Defensiveness in Adults.' *American Journal of Occupational Therapy 49*, 5, 444–451.

Koenig, K. (2003) 'Behavioral Responsiveness: The Relationship Between Temperament and Sensory Processing.' Paper presented at the American Occupational Therapy Association National Meeting, Washington, DC.

Linderman, T.M. and Stewart, K.B. (1999) 'Sensory Integrative-based Occupational Therapy and Functional Outcomes in Young Children with Pervasive Developmental Disorders: A Single-subject Study.' *American Journal of Occupational Therapy 53*, 2, 207–213.

McIntosh, D., Miller, L., Shyu, V. and Hagerman, R. (1999) 'Sensory Modulation Disruption, Electrodermal Responses and Functional Behaviors.' *Developmental Medicine and Child Neurology 41*, 9, 608–615.

Miguel, E.C., Do Rosario-Campos, M.C., da Silva Prado, H., Do Valle, R., Rauch, S.L., Coffey, B.J. *et al.* (2000) 'Sensory Phenomena in Obsessive-compulsive Disorder and Tourette's Disorder.' *Journal of Clinical Psychiatry 61*, 2, 150–156.

Miller, L., McIntosh, D., McGrath, J., Shyu, V., Lampe, M., Taylor, A. *et al.* (1998) 'Electrodermal Responses to Sensory Stimuli in Individuals with Fragile X Syndrome: A Preliminary Report.' *American Journal of Medical Genetics 83*, 4, 268–279.

Parham, L.D. (1998) 'The Relationship of Sensory Integrative Development to Achievement in Elementary Students: Four-Year Longitudinal Patterns.' *Occupational Therapy Journal of Research 18*, 3, 105–127.

Provost, B. and Oetter, P. (1993) 'The Sensory Rating Scale for Infants and Young Children: Development and Reliability.' *Physical and Occupational Therapy in Pediatrics 13*, 4, 15–35.

Schaaf, R.C., Miller, L.J., Sewell, D. and O'Keefe, S. (2003) 'Preliminary Study of Parasympathetic Functioning in Children with Sensory Modulation Dysfunction and its Relation to Occupation.' *American Journal of Occupational Therapy 57*, 4, 442–449.

Shumway-Cook, A. and Woollacott, M. (2000) 'Attentional Demands and Postural Control: The Effect of Sensory Context.' *Journal of Gerontology: Medical Sciences 55A*, 1, M10–M16.

Smith-Roley, S., Blanche, E. and Schaaf, R.C. (eds) (2001) *The Nature of Sensory Integration with Diverse Populations.* Tucson, AZ: Psychological Corporation.

Stephens, C.L. and Royeen, C.B. (1998) 'Investigation of Tactile Defensiveness and Self-esteem in Typically Developing Children.' *Occupational Therapy International 5*, 4, 273–280.

Tickle-Degnen, L. and Coster, W. (1995) 'Therapeutic Interaction and the Management of Challenge During the Beginning Minutes of Sensory Integration Treatment.' *Occupational Therapy Journal of Research 15*, 2, 122–141.

Watling, R. (1998) 'Selected Literature Exploring the Effectiveness of a Sensory-based Approach to the Treatment of Autism.' *Physical and Occupational Therapy in Pediatrics 18,* 2, 77–85.

Wiener, A.S., Long, T., DeGangi, G. and Battaile, B. (1996) 'Sensory Processing of Infants Born Prematurely or with Regulatory Disorders.' *Physical and Occupational Therapy in Pediatrics 16,* 4, 1–17.

Zuckerman, M. (1993) 'Out of Sensory Deprivation and into Sensation Seeking: A Personal and Scientific Journey.' In G.G. Brannigan and M.R. Merrens (eds) *The Undaunted Psychologist: Adventures in Research.* Philadelphia: Temple University Press.